KW-051-158

Department of Child Health
The Queen's University of Belfast

Clinics in Developmental Medicine No. 130
RUNNING A TEAM FOR DISABLED CHILDREN
AND THEIR FAMILIES

© 1994 Mac Keith Press
526/529 High Holborn House, 52–54 High Holborn, London WC1V 6RL

All rights reserved. No part of this publication may be reproduced, stored in a retrieval system, or transmitted in any form or by any means, electronic, mechanical, photocopying, recording or otherwise, without the prior permission of the publishers

First published in this edition 1994

British Library Cataloguing-in-Publication data:
A catalogue record for this book is available from the British Library

ISSN: 0069 4835
ISBN: 0 901260 99 1

Printed in Great Britain at The Lavenham Press Ltd., Lavenham, Suffolk
Mac Keith Press is supported by **The Spastics Society, London, England**

Clinics in Developmental Medicine No. 130

Running a Team for Disabled Children & their Families

MARTIN F. ROBARDS

Children's Department
Pembury Hospital
Tunbridge Wells, Kent

1994
Mac Keith Press

Distributed by CAMBRIDGE
UNIVERSITY PRESS

To Julie

AUTHOR'S APPOINTMENT

MARTIN ROBARDS,
BSc, FRCP

Consultant Paediatrician, Children's Department,
Pembury Hospital, Pembury, Tunbridge Wells, Kent

CONTENTS

FOREWORD

Children with special developmental, medical or educational needs constitute approximately 20 per cent of the child population in many countries of the Western world. A wide variety of disorders cause or contribute to these needs, and as a result services, particularly in the medical community, have traditionally been organized independently along diagnostic lines. Thus, for example, the cerebral palsy clinic often operates separately from the spina bifida programme, and both are usually distinct from services offered to children with mental handicaps or learning disabilities. In many places these services actually constitute multiple disparate teams and approaches, even within a single community or institution.

In this text, Martin Robards offers a thought provoking set of ideas about the organization, constitution, mandate and activities of a local team for disabled children and their families. His point of departure is his experience of almost two decades working as a community-based developmental paediatrician in south-east England. There the services have evolved as he and his group have approached and resolved complex issues concerning the delivery of specialized medical, educational, developmental and social services to children with developmental disabilities and their families. Although Martin Robards' roots are English, the concepts he has developed in this book are broad and applicable generally, the references eclectic and international.

At first glance the thought of reading (let alone writing) such a book might seem a recipe for terminal boredom! We all *know* what is needed for 'these children', and how to do it. We know why we do what we do, and with what goals . . . or do we? After a careful reading of this text I found myself repeatedly challenged about the assumptions we make in the daily activities of our own developmental services. As a visitor to programmes outside my community, I always find it much easier to question the basis of what my hosts are telling me than to sit back and reflect on the goals and operations of the things we do at home.

This is a book written by a clinician for clinicians. Its value lies in the challenges it poses to each reader to think about their own ways of dealing with the clinical and structural aspects of services for children with disabilities and their families. How do we handle these various clinical problems in our community? How do we think about 'disability' and 'handicap', and what implications do these concepts have for what we do? What models guide our thinking and our service organization? Who do we not serve, and why not? These and other questions will certainly occur to any attentive reader. Far from being a parochial account of 'how we do it', the text covers a range of related aspects of services for disabled children, with a thoughtful exploration of many of the relevant considerations that should be part of planning and implementing services. Models are presented and discussed, with useful references to additional reading. Furthermore, the author bravely commits to paper his team's approach to many of the thorny problems that inevitably challenge any group providing a range of consultation, assessment, treatment and follow-up services for the wide array of children served by programmes like Dr Robards'. However, this is not a set of standards or guidelines for service organization. We are never given the message that this is the way things must be done.

The book's Introduction provides a background about teams for disabled children, describing the evolution of services in the UK to the current organization of services for these populations. Chapter 1 uses a variety of case illustrations—both 'typical' cases described in an idealized manner, and 'real life' experiences of Dr Robards' team—to set the tone for the book by outlining the complexities faced by professionals who work with disabled children and their families. The 'cases taken from real experience' are particularly useful because the reader is given an insight into the thinking of the clinicians who dealt with the issues described, and learns about failures as well as successes in implementing the assessment and management strategies described in the ensuing chapters. Among other features of these case vignettes, one is exposed to the range of problems referred to the team for disabled children, and can begin to recognize the commonalities across a range of developmental disorders and disabilities.

Chapter 2 offers an introduction to terminology commonly heard in the field of disability. There is a logic to these concepts, and their appropriate usage is discussed. Although the author is too polite to say so, the message from this chapter is that consistent application of these terms and the concepts that underlie them would both sharpen our discourse with one another, and consolidate some of these concepts beyond their current liberal and often inconsistent usage.

In Chapter 3 Robards outlines epidemiological findings from studies in Canada, the UK and the Nordic countries, to remind the reader of the scope of neuro-developmental disorders and related chronic problems. In the context of a defined geographical and population base for a service (such as is possible where services are regionally allocated in a somewhat rational manner), it is possible to calculate approximate rates of various types of disabling conditions, and to plan services accordingly. Furthermore, it should then be possible to compare a programme's prevalence figures with those calculated for the district (which are almost always higher), and to institute measures to find children whose needs could be met by these services if they were referred. In fact, there is some discussion about the value of knowing about all the potentially eligible children in a district, but the reader is left to consider individually the costs in time and effort to achieve such a goal. (In North America and other parts of the world, health care delivery is less co-ordinated centrally, and under these circumstances it may be much more difficult to know what portion of the population one's services are being asked to see, unless these services are the only specialty programmes in the area.)

In many ways Chapter 4 is the most challenging section of the book. As Robards illustrates with both text and schematics, the structure and function of a child disability team can take many forms, with a wide variety of styles of operation. Here as much as anywhere the reader is forced to reflect on how these activities are organized and provided in their own community, and to consider what assumptions underlie that particular pattern of team function. For this reader, at least, these issues provoke more debate and consume more energy than almost any others at our clinic. Issues of territoriality, trust, leadership, ownership . . . all are touched on, gently but firmly, either in the text or between the lines. This chapter should probably be read and discussed together by all members of any team, perhaps with each member drawing their 'artist's conception' of team structure as outlined at the end of the chapter.

Is a Child Development Centre really necessary? In Chapter 5 the author discusses some of the considerations that form an answer to this question. A number of useful arguments are offered in favour of a 'bricks and mortar' facility around which to focus service activities. These ideas will be especially helpful to clinicians whose hospital administrators believe that closing the facility in favour of 'community-based' services is rational!

Chapter 6 explores issues and activities involved in the consultation process, including some thoughts about the potential therapeutic benefit to parents of an effective consultation. It is always interesting to learn how a fellow clinician approaches a familiar activity like an initial consultation, and the outline of ideas and models offered here is rich in clinically useful thinking. Thus, for example, the venue and style of a first assessment (general paediatric clinic or Child Development Centre) will be guided to some degree by the nature and apparent severity of the presenting problem(s). Referral to other members of the assessment team is not automatic, but rather is predicated upon the developmentalist's judgement about the need for further clinical assessment information. Furthermore, pre-assessment planning can follow the initial paediatric consultation, so that the team may take full advantage of information about the child already available in the community, but not yet in hand.

The actual process of the consultation is outlined with sensitivity and valuable insights. Robards highlights several of the common themes involved in addressing and answering parents' questions—What is it? Why did it happen? What about the future? What can be done? Will it recur? These queries are predictable, and answers can often be formulated (in plain language) with the expectation that these will form the kernel of the conversation.

Several styles of consultation are reviewed, and as elsewhere in this book, these should provoke thought and discussion among team members who read the book together. It is clear that there have been major shifts in the doctor–patient relationship over the past two decades, such that the way in which (in the 90's lingo) 'health professionals' 'interact' with 'clients' is vastly different from the traditional 'expert' doctor model. Readers should consider the implications of each of the several models of consultation discussed in this chapter, both in order to discover their own preferred style, and to recognize the implications for service delivery that each model implies. (It is worth noting here that Robards has looked at models in the developing world as well as those from the West, and one suspects that there is much to learn from the ideas to which he alludes in passing.)

What happens after the consultation has produced a formulation about the nature, extent and meaning of a child's problems? Chapter 7 discusses a variety of challenges involved in follow-up and referrals for additional assessments and second opinions. Reference is made to some of the thorny ethical dilemmas faced by a team, such as when parents choose not to follow through with appointments, or when tensions arise between parents and professionals, or when parents want a second opinion. There are some good suggestions about how joint consultations with other specialists can be facilitated, or referrals made to trusted colleagues and services thought to be more relevant to the needs of child and family than one's own. A particularly uncomfortable issue concerns transfer of services for the graduates of our child development programmes, whose needs persist despite outgrowing the services developed for young people. In many communities this transition remains an incompletely resolved dilemma.

Chapter 8 reviews evidence concerning what parents want from social services and health professionals, referring to studies from both sides of the Atlantic that address a variety of perspectives. The major section of the chapter focuses on therapies, both traditional and alternative approaches, that are generally available to families with a child with a disability. Key issues include the value of 'early intervention', and the usefulness of the Portage Programme with which Robards' group has considerable experience. In this chapter (as well as briefly in Chapter 7) there is discussion of 'alternative' and innovative therapies of uncertain reputation or value, with some wise thoughts about ways to help parents understand these approaches in the context of what is already offered to them in 'standard' care and services. There is also a plea for more and better evaluation of everything we do.

The final two chapters discuss the importance of education—of the team, community colleagues, junior health professionals, parents and the public—and of liaison and communication across the many sectors of the community. There are references to models of record keeping, including case registers, and discussion of parents' access to their child's and family's notes. Once again the reader will be forced to think about what they do to address the issues these chapters discuss, especially in a changing world of parents' rights, access to information, and confidentiality.

All developmental clinicians owe Dr Robards their thanks. By aggregating in a single book an important set of ideas, experiences and reflections about running a service for children with disabilities and their families, he has provided us with a valuable resource. Far from being the last word on these subjects (each chapter could be expanded into a text of its own), this book is an insightful beginning—a challenge to thoughtful practitioners to review what we do, to study variations of these many themes, and to add new knowledge about the how and what of our day-to-day practices. By sharing our experiences, dilemmas and scholarly ideas in the way this book has done, we all can contribute to move the field forward, and to improve the quality of life of children with disabilities and their families.

PETER ROSENBAUM, M.D., F.R.C.P.(C)
Director of Paediatrics
Chedoke Child and Family Centre
Chedoke–McMaster Hospitals
Hamilton, Ontario, Canada

INTRODUCTION: BACKGROUND AND EVOLUTION

Background

There is a group of children whose disabilities are such that they demand a different kind of service from that required by most children attending paediatric clinics. These children and their families need a service which is flexible and adaptable to their needs as well as being comprehensive. This does not exclude or substitute for other statutory and voluntary services already available to them in areas of health care, education and social support.

At one end of the spectrum there is the child with multiple disabilities, complex neurological problems or physical problems compounded by psychological and behavioural difficulties: most paediatricians would agree that such children need an approach somewhat different from that of an ordinary paediatric consultation.

At the other end of the spectrum there are children with disabilities falling into the same category of disorder, but with a lower level of severity, *e.g.* a mild hemiplegia, reasonably controlled epilepsy or situation-specific over-activity. For these children the paediatrician, in consultation with the parents and sometimes other specialists on a one-off basis, can offer the necessary diagnostic consultation and interventions in a conventional manner without much need for interdisciplinary activity.

Between these two ends of the spectrum is a third group of children who will sometimes require reviews by a team of professionals with complementary skills and experience, while at other times the child and his or her family might best be dealt with by just one member of the group.

It may be that all children with a neurodevelopmental problem should be seen at least once by the Team for Disabled Children and their Families (TDC), for reasons that will be discussed later.

In the UK there is a hierarchy for referral. The general practitioners (GPs), who are true generalists (despite the advice of the Court Report (1976) for some of them to become general practitioner paediatricians), refer on to general paediatricians in district general hospitals. This is the secondary referral level. Tertiary referral, usually at regional level, is to paediatric neurologists, developmental paediatricians and other specialists.

In North America specialisation tends to occur at an earlier level, and whereas in the UK there are community paediatricians and clinical medical officers working in parallel with the hospital paediatricians and engaging in child health and developmental surveillance, in North America this is mostly done by developmental paediatricians at the secondary or tertiary level of referral.

In the UK there is very little private practice in paediatrics and even less in childhood disability. This means that those who work in this field are not encumbered by considerations of the cost of a consultation in terms of the time taken by the child and family, or the 'opportunity costs' of being unable to see other children during that time.

In North America, patients represent income to practitioners who may consequently be reluctant to refer on or to share the care with others unless there is an overwhelming necessity so to do. Rosenbaum (1987) also refers to non-billable medical work under provincial health plans which create fiscal tensions.

Problems may be encountered in getting professionals to disengage from patients who would be better managed by some other person or group of people. This is not only a problem of reward but also of priorities: for example, a baby with Down syndrome may be followed up by the general paediatrician and paediatric cardiologist even though the baby's main requirement is in the area of early intervention and stimulation for psychomotor delay. Often the level of activity around the physical problem will lead to the other needs being unrecognised, or recognised but unmet.

Not only may the needs of the child go unrecognised but even more frequently the needs of families, and assessment of the kind of help they require, may be overlooked by the lone professional attempting to provide for all their needs. One might make a case for a team approach where the child's problem is unipolar but where other problems within the family are so complex that a straightforward approach to the child's difficulties would not be beneficial.

Another aspect of the team approach is one of personality and empathy between parents and professionals. Despite the fact that many parents find having three or four professionals at one consultation initially difficult to deal with, it does give them the opportunity to identify the person with whom they can communicate best, especially if there have been difficulties with the individual to whom they had previously been linked. Similarly, the team approach may give families the feeling that they are getting an automatic second opinion and a fresh approach to their problems.

When TDCs were first set up in the UK, they were known as District Handicap Teams (DHTs). The initiative for them usually came from the health authority, either the community medical officers or paediatricians, and although a tripartite system incorporating education, social services and health was recommended in the Court Report (1976), the social services and health elements were mostly introduced at a later date. The Court Report (paras. 14.23 and 14.24) envisaged that:

14.23   The team would have two distinct functions, one clinical and the other operational. The clinical function would be:
  i to provide investigation and assessment of certain individual children with complex disorders and to arrange and co-ordinate their treatment;
  ii to provide their parents, teachers, child care staff, and others who may be directly concerned in their care, with the professional advice and support that can guide them in their management of the children;
  iii to encourage and assist professional field-work staff in their management and surveillance of these and other handicapped children locally, by being available for consultation either in the district child development centre . . . or in local premises;
  iv to provide primary and supporting specialist services to special schools in the district.

14.24   The operational functions would be:
  i to be involved with others at district and area level in epidemiological surveys of need; to monitor the effectiveness of the district service for handicapped children; to present data and

suggestions for the development of the service; and to maintain the quality of its institutions;

ii to act as source of information in the district about handicap in children and the services available;

iii to organise seminars and courses of training for professional staff working in the district.

In their 1985 report on DHTs, Bax and Whitmore found that 82 of the 192 district health authorities in the UK had DHTs and assessment centres; and 32 health authorities had in addition a DHT without an assessment centre. The constitution and functions of these teams varied enormously and some had only their titles in common. Nevertheless there may be benefits in this diversity and in allowing the evolution of such teams in geographically distinct areas which have unique populations and particular strengths and weaknesses in existing services, rather than imposing a standardised formula on every health authority to provide a service which might not be entirely appropriate. Thus, if a service evolves under the supervision of local professionals who know the strengths and weaknesses of the existing service, one should finish with few gaps, little duplication and a more efficient and effective service. This of course assumes that there are no vested interests other than the provision of a reasonable level of service for the children and their families, that there is no unprofessional blocking of service provision and that financial support is adequate and secure.

What happened before we had teams for disabled children? Sometimes nothing very different, but there was a tendency for more children to be managed at the tertiary level. Recommendations were often made at that level in ignorance of local services such as special schools. Management at tertiary level usually had a cost in travel for parents and caused uncertainties because of the remoteness of the service. Often children and parents muddled along together not realising what other services were available for them locally because those services were conducted in isolation and there was no system to span the statutory and voluntary sectors. It was more usual to have a request for information from an agency than to receive a report from one, a situation that is now reversed.

A criticism sometimes levelled at TDCs is that responsibility for the patient is ambiguous. This is not so; each professional has his or her own responsibilities in the same way as if all consultations were being conducted on a one-to-one basis. It is mainly information, not responsibility, which is being shared. This is demonstrated to parents with each joint consultation where team work is shown to be real and not imaginary.

Evolution

TDCs have mostly evolved through the enthusiasm of a few participants and encouragement from the statutory and voluntary organisations. That is how it happened in my own health authority.

Beginning 18 years ago as a newly appointed paediatrician, I found that I was seeing in general clinics a number of children whose problems were more time consuming than most, with psychosocial effects on the family which were more handicapping than one might have predicted on the basis of the child's primary diagnosis. Some of these children had common paediatric conditions such as diabetes mellitus or asthma with severe psychological problems or family dysfunction, but the majority had neurodevelopmental disorders. For the former, help was traditionally available through the child and family psychiatric service or hospital medical social worker, but for the latter one felt that the evolving neurodevelopmental problem dictated that the paediatrician should take the major role because usually the diagnosis and prognosis would remain in question for some time.

It was therefore rational for the paediatrician to draw supporting professionals closer to the family/paediatric interface, and gradually joint consultations with the medical social worker, senior clinical medical officer, physiotherapist, and psychologist evolved. The evolution of the team depends on who can help, and not necessarily on professional qualifications or disciplines. The personality of the individual appears to be more important to the family than professional background. Sloper and Turner (1992) also found that the combination of openness, honesty in giving information and patience in listening to parents was what parents of children with severe physical disability most valued in professionals. Similarly, Rosenbaum (1987) found that the 'functions' of the individual team member were more important than his or her professional background .

Once the team has been formed, there are dangers of 'over-structuring'. There is a risk of institutionalisation and loss of the personal approach and approachability. Ferlie *et al.* (1984) in a survey of services for mentally handicapped people in the South East Thames Regional Health Authority give a clear example of this. Most UK health authorities have set up Community Mental Handicap Teams (CMHTs)—sometimes now known as Community Learning Disability Teams—over the last 15 years. These teams offer the services of specialist nurses, social workers, therapists and medical officers. Their style tends to be based on a 'social model' rather than the 'medical model' adopted by most teams for disabled children or TDCs. The National Development Group for the Mentally Handicapped (1977) described the CMHTs initially as a way of supporting children (and adults) with their families in the community and keeping them out of long-stay institutional care.

Ferlie *et al.* found that the vast majority of parents had never heard of the CMHTs and suggested that the teams were too inward looking and should correct this by, for example, accepting referrals from anyone. They said that there is a danger that complicated structures for joint working not only absorb valuable professional time, but also make it harder for clients to grasp how the service actually works. They encouraged the identification of key workers and written information to describe the function of these teams.

Thus we can see that accessibility depends on contact with a person who may be a member of the team, but not necessarily with 'the team'. Therefore responsibilities within the team for taking referrals and liaising with other members must be established and nurtured.

It is also clear from basic child care practice, but not always to the helping professionals, that though the child is the patient, the consumer of the service is the family. It therefore follows that the family predicament or the child's environment will determine the type of service required rather than just the narrow consideration of the child's pathology. In our own (unpublished) survey of parents' perceptions of our Portage service (see Chapter 8) it was clear that their own needs were as important, or more important, to the family than the primary needs of the child. Therefore the service to the child must be designed within the context of the family.

Another stage of the development of the team and its service is the realisation that non-medical people group neurodevelopmental problems into levels of physical, intellectual and other abilities rather than using medical diagnostic groups and that they take what could be described as a non-categorical approach. It is often surprising to the paediatrician that children can be admitted to educational establishments and institutional care with very explicit evaluations of their physical, intellectual and emotional abilities, but with no clue as to the underlying medical diagnosis, if indeed one has been reached. Paediatricians feel uncomfortable with this and need to explore the background to be sure that at least the issue of progressive disease and the genetic aspects of the case have been fully examined.

Nevertheless, paediatricians and others who are committed to the medical diagnosis and medical management of a case may be in a minority when the total service load attributable to the family of a child with a psychomotor problem is calculated. Perhaps we should be more aware of how others see and classify the needs of children and their families than we are at present. Bailey *et al.* (1993) have recently shown that a system to describe functional ability and disability in children can achieve a high level of reliability between ratings performed by professionals of different disciplines and parents.

If we accept that the majority of people caring for children with neurodevelopmental problems are parents or non-health working professionals, then who should judge the effectiveness or otherwise of the interventions instituted by the TDC? Should it be done by peer group review of the TDC or by a process of analysis of customer satisfaction or by a combination of both? As health care resources become more limited, this function will assume greater importance.

Finally, the TDC exists to evaluate, inform and advise, and should be regarded as a system for enabling change in the child and his or her immediate environment.

REFERENCES

Bailey, D.B., Simeonsson, R.J., Buysse, V., Smith, T. (1993) 'Reliability of an index of child characteristics.' *Developmental Medicine and Child Neurology*, **35**, 806-815.
Bax, M.C.O., Whitmore, K. (1985) *District Handicap Teams: Structure, Function and Relationships. Report to DHSS.* London: Community Paediatric Research Unit, Westminster Children's Hospital.
Court Report (1976) *Fit for the Future. Report of the Committee on Child Health Services. Vol. 1. Cmnd. 6684.* London: HMSO.
Ferlie, E., Pahl, J., Quine, L. (1984) 'Professional collaboration in services for mentally handicapped people.' *Journal for Social Policy*, **13**, 185-202.
National Development Group for the Mentally Handicapped (1977) *Mentally Handicapped Children: a Plan for Action. Pamphlet No.2.* London: DHSS.
Rosenbaum P. (1987) 'Children with chronic handicaps: implications for care giving.' *In:* Tonkin R.S., Wright J.R. (Eds.) *Redesigning Relationships in Child Health Care. Proceedings of a Symposium held February 20–21, 1987.* Vancouver: British Columbia Children's Hospital.
Sloper, P., Turner, S. (1992) 'Service Needs of Families of Children with Severe Physical Disability.' *Child: Care, Health and Development*, **18**, 259-282

1
CRITICAL PATHWAYS FOR SOME DIFFICULT CASES

In this chapter I am going to describe some individual cases and families with which TDCs have to deal. The first half consists of four typical cases to illustrate the scope of work of the TDC, with different children having different types of problems. These cases are described in a somewhat theoretical and idealised manner to indicate what might be the evolution of the problem and its implications, in terms of therapy and other interventions.

The second half of the chapter summarises the biographies of seven real families, three of them having more than one child with problems relevant to the TDC. These families demonstrate how much more complex these management problems become in practice compared with the theoretical cases. They also demonstrate the need to consider the total environment and 'ecology' of the child and the family rather than merely the pathology and natural history of the child's affliction.

Typical theoretical cases
A baby with fits and hypotonia from the neonatal intensive care unit (NICU)
A sick infant being discharged from the NICU illustrates the difficulties of hand-over from an acute medical environment to the service of long term follow-up and therapy. The baby's problems will hinge to some extent on whether a definitive diagnosis has already been reached. The possibilities are numerous. At one end of the scale there may be a single unifying diagnosis with a clear cause which is well understood and well explained to the parents. At the other end of the scale, which will include many approximations of a diagnosis and cause, there may be no adequate explanation of the problem even after extensive investigation. The state of knowledge about the child and the parents' understanding of that knowledge—or ignorance—will have a major impact on the subsequent course of events. Such a child and family will need anti-convulsant therapy and its monitoring; physiotherapy; possibly an early intervention programme; and social work support. Follow-up is usually fairly frequent to begin with. Often fits are difficult to control, and the neurodevelopmental status is at its most dynamic phase of evolution in the first few months. Depending on diagnosis, there may be a need to involve a clinical geneticist, a paediatric neurologist and other specialists in management. At this early phase parental expectations are usually being established and it is important to explore these and give early guidance concerning their level of realism.

Outcome for these babies covers a very wide spectrum and many investigations and assessments may be necessary before a clear rate of progress is evident. It is easy to concentrate too much on the mechanics and anatomy of the child and overlook the functional aspects. If s/he is a first child the parents may have entirely-inappropriate models of normal child development and not appreciate how their baby deviates from the norm. Often parents need to be given time to realise the extent of the problem, and it is counter-productive to work too actively against blocking or denial at this stage.

A baby with Down syndrome
When a baby is recognised shortly after birth as having Down syndrome, the position is very different from that described above. There is a wealth of knowledge concerning how the process of informing the parents about the child should be conducted (Cunningham *et al.* 1984, Quine and Pahl 1987). Furthermore the prognosis has reasonably defined limits and allows one to be optimistic that 'normal' schooling may be a possibility for the child and that a healthy childhood can be contemplated. It is not generally helpful to go into too much detail at the first interview concerning all the possible complications associated with the syndrome. In practice the clinical examination, with a normal ECG and echocardiogram should rule out most associated congenital abnormalities (Tubman *et al.* 1991). If the total picture is obvious, it is not helpful to hedge your bets by saying that you won't be sure about the diagnosis until chromosome results are available. But genetic counselling later and prenatal diagnosis in subsequent pregnancies will hinge on the chromosome findings. Early contact with a parent support group should be offered and often it will be necessary for this to be arranged on behalf of the parents whose ability to initiate such contact may well be inhibited by their state of shock.

The major problems for Down syndrome babies and their follow-up in the Child Development Centre (CDC) are that those who have congenital heart disease or other anomalies requiring acute medical intervention tend to come into the system late and have their psychomotor problems overlooked initially. It is useful to develop a referral system to ensure that the acute specialist care does not block access to early intervention programmes and other TDC services.

Follow-up for these children later needs to include periodic testing of vision and hearing, thyroid function tests (Selikowitz 1993), and possibly X-ray of the cervical spine for atlanto-axial instability if they wish to indulge in certain sports, although the value of this is debatable (Selby *et al.* 1991, Cremers *et al.* 1993). Often Down syndrome children and their families demand very little of the TDC, and sometimes the team needs to adopt a role as advocate for the child if the parents take a too non-interventionist approach. This, of course, may be true of children with other disabilities.

Follow-up for these children can be conducted by the medical officers in the schools that the children attend, and the TDC input may be very low later on, but the Community Learning Disability Team (CLDT) will need to become involved in the teenage years to ensure that housing, employment and other issues are addressed.

A child with diplegia
The age at which a child with diplegia presents for diagnosis depends upon at least two factors: firstly, the severity of the disability, and secondly, whether there are predisposing

factors such as extreme prematurity. Some children with no predisposing factors and a mild disability, perhaps with parents who are not perceptive, may not reach medical attention until well into their schooling, particularly if they attend a school where there are no routine medical examinations. However, in children presenting late, an hereditary form of spastic paraplegia should be considered (Gordon 1993).

Usually, however, the difficulties of gait will be apparent in the first year or two of life. For children being followed up from a NICU there will be a high level of suspicion, and if psychomotor development deviates from the norm, the diagnosis can be made over a series of attendances. Thus the concepts of disability and cerebral palsy can be gradually introduced to the parents.

The child who presents with no predisposing factor but who is late in walking or has an abnormal gait brings rather different problems. Diagnosis here may well come as a severe shock to the parents and it needs to be dealt with in a sensitive and constructive manner. Often these children will be brought to the clinic by the mother alone, and an early follow up arrangement to see both parents, together with other members of the TDC (*e.g.* a physiotherapist and a social worker), can be helpful in getting problems into perspective and providing the family with early expert support.

When the diagnosis of diplegia is secure and the implications have been explained, it is time to consider the genetic implications. Before raising the issue I always ask parents about their plans for further children. It is important to know the difference between the parents having no immediate plans and one or both of them having been sterilised. In the former case genetic advice can be arranged at the parents' convenience and in the latter it will probably be unnecessary, except perhaps for the brothers and sisters. It is equally important to ask, if appropriate, whether the mother could be pregnant at that moment because if she is, the issue will require very sensitive handling and more urgent advice.

These principles, of course, apply whenever exploring genetic issues with parents. The general public is on the whole unaware of the genetic implications of cerebral palsy and many doctors share this ignorance. When there is a symmetrical form of cerebral palsy without obvious prenatal or postnatal causation, the likelihood of recurrence is of the order of one in eight to one in ten. About half of those cases probably represent autosomal recessive inheritance, the others being sporadic (Hughes and Newton 1992). Referral to a clinical geneticist, with full information about the circumstances, should help give the parents an objective view of their prospects for further pregnancies.

The diplegic child always requires regular physiotherapy supervision, and often the therapist will be the link person with the child's school or preschool nursery. It is usually the therapist's job to initiate and supervise orthotics and walking aids.

Of children with cerebral palsy, the diplegic child is more likely than any other to be helped by combined consultations between the TDC members and orthopaedic surgeons. This is especially so if a gait laboratory or at least some objective gait analysis system is available. The science of gait analysis should now allow, indeed encourage, outcome analysis of orthopaedic interventions in children with cerebral palsy. This should promote clinical audit of such interventions as routine, rather than just for research purposes (Gage 1992).

A child with a neurodegenerative condition

Of all the problems with which parents may have to cope, a child with progressive neuro-logical degeneration is one of the most stressful and difficult. These are uncommon diseases, but a significant amount of a TDC's work will be with the families of children with rare neurological syndromes, some of which will be progressive degenerative disorders.

Sometimes in older children the period between initial symptoms and the confirmation of a definite diagnosis can be quite lengthy. Several opinions may have been sought and many investigations performed before the diagnosis, prognosis and genetic implications become clear. The whole process, combined with the immediate effects on the family of the child's loss of intellect, mobility and awareness, can be devastating. Much practical support to help with the family's physical, financial and emotional needs is required. There will be many professionals and others involved with such a family, and identifying a named person or key worker in such a situation helps focus and co-ordinate activities and services and provides an advocate through whom the parents can act.

There is often a protracted grieving process, especially when it is an older child who has already developed identity, personality and a group of friends who begins gradually and inexorably to deteriorate in intellect and physique. Inexperienced staff may not realise how painful this process can be and what a sense of relief is felt by the family and those intimately involved with them when the child eventually dies. The role of the TDC must be one of support, not only for the family, recognising the different needs of the parents, brothers and sisters, but also for other individuals who have been involved with the family and are touched by the loss.

When the end comes, a review of such cases by the TDC will reveal good practice and shortcomings. This provides a relatively sensitive measure of the effectiveness and efficiency of the team. It should be possible to identify critical incidents, both positive and negative, in the management of a patient so that practice can be modified for other families. Outcome measures in traditional health terms are largely irrelevant, and criteria for good practice should be defined by peer group reviews.

Cases taken from real experience

Readers who are involved as TDC members will be able to recall various children and families who highlight the principles of good practice because they have availed themselves of the various services offered by the TDC and have been perceived as benefiting from those services. Experienced team members will also recall other children and families where management has not been ideal and where problems have arisen in various ways. Some of these families and children have complex problems and some are more straightforward. I describe below some children and families who demonstrate the variety of difficulties posed to the team by straightforward pathology and by complex pathology. These cases show how the attitudes of families and their interactions with the team influence the style of service which they receive, and the variety of ways in which attempts are made to help. These attempts are not always successful so I have tried to illustrate short-comings and failures of the service as well as successes.

A baby with progressive neurological disease

In this example the role of the team is to provide material and emotional support to the child and family. The former may mean ensuring that the physical needs of the child are met and that the home environment is adapted as necessary. The latter may require the provision of respite care, for both the physical and psychological relief of the parents. Also, members of the team need to demonstrate that they understand the anxieties and fears that parents have of their child's physical, intellectual and psychological disintegration. The special skills of individual team members in providing support may be based more on their own personality and style than on their specific professional training. It is likely that key workers will be identified from the team through whom communications between the family, the team and other agencies will be channelled.

Matthew was first brought to see me when he was 13 months of age. He had been investigated at a tertiary referral centre because he had been hypotonic from six weeks of age and had developed infantile spasms at six months. Investigations at that time included chromosome analysis, cerebral computed tomography (CT) scan and magnetic resonance imaging (MRI). His electromyogram (EMG) had shown a severe myopathy, and muscle biopsy had shown a lipid storage disorder. The other investigations were normal and his fits improved with ACTH therapy. The therapy was continued for three months and Matthew was subsequently treated with clonazepam and phenobarbitone.

A specific diagnosis of Matthew's problem was not made at this stage, but it appeared that he had a severe lipid storage disorder which was not only inhibiting his motor development but also having a severe effect on his intellectual capacity. His parents were advised by the geneticist that it was highly likely that this condition was inherited as an autosomal recessive disorder and the implications of this were explained in some detail.

Matthew's management centred around instructing his mother in physiotherapy, giving her support and, because he accumulated oral secretions and had a very poor cough reflex, supplying her with one electric sucker for home use and a portable one as well. He also needed management for severe constipation.

Further support was provided through the team medical social worker who put the parents in touch with other families of severely disabled children, and informed them of statutory allowances. She gave them our local booklet concerning statutory and voluntary services for special needs children, including all the local and national elements, and finally she introduced Matthew to our local home-based early intervention programme (Portage—see Chapter 8). Matthew also needed regular reviews to monitor his anticonvulsant therapy.

Because he was so disabled and required fairly skilled nursing care from his mother, it was important to admit him to the children's ward at the local hospital for holiday periods and when his parents wanted to have a break for weeks or weekends, and this was done on a regular basis.

Eighteen months after Matthew's birth, his mother told us that she was pregnant again, following AID (artificial insemination by donor) therapy. During this pregnancy Matthew required tube feeding because of severe swallowing problems and enemas because of his constipation. Several admissions were arranged for him during that time.

After his brother was born, a link family was organised who looked after Matthew from time to time on a prearranged basis, receiving from the parents tokens which subsequently were cashed in with the social services department.

Matthew died on the children's ward aged four years and an autopsy was arranged at the tertiary referral centre where his initial investigations had been performed. The final diagnosis was one of dentato-olivary dysplasia. The consensus of genetic opinion was that this was a sporadic problem although a recessive mode of inheritance could not be completely ruled out. Matthew's brother was developing completely normally and there was no doubt that he was unaffected by the disease. The family have planned no further children.

I visited the parents at home after Matthew's death and subsequently wrote to them concerning the post-mortem examination reports. Because they had been very much involved with his management and kept informed of all the investigations, they found it easier to cope with his death than had it been sudden and unexpected. They demonstrated their gratitude to the unit by donating a substantial sum of money which they had collected from well-wishers (this helped us to fund a soft play area in the CDC).

While the inexorable decline in the abilities of a child and the ultimate death of that child are seen in traditional medical terms as failure, in many ways Matthew's management was rewarding for those who sought to help because his parents were responsive to the support they were given. They worked with us as a team, we shared their anxieties and grief and they were able to demonstrate their gratitude in a practical way after Matthew's death.

A baby with hydrocephalus

The next child also died, but the sequence of events was rather different from that of the previous boy. Michael was making progress, then had a severe setback. His parents tried desperately to help him, struggling against severe odds, but eventually he died. In this case the TDC only became involved after a child with an initially good prognosis suffered severe complications at a tertiary referral centre. We were dealing with parents who were already very disappointed and angry about the management of their child. We failed to achieve optimum working relationships, but with compromise on both sides some members of the team were able to contribute practical support.

Michael was the second baby of healthy professional parents. He was born following caesarean section: there had been failure to progress in labour, non-engagement of the head and polyhydramnios. His hydrocephalus had not been diagnosed prenatally but was obvious at birth, his head circumference measuring 46 cm. He was transferred to a neuro-surgical unit directly after birth and had a ventriculo-peritoneal shunt inserted without event. The CT scan suggested there might be a venous malformation causing aqueductal stenosis which had led to hydrocephalus.

Michael's progress thereafter was satisfactory, and at four months it was noticed that a small amount of cerebrospinal fluid (CSF) was collecting under the scalp, around the site of the shunt, and that he had developed several dermal haemangiomas. His head circumference, growth and psychomotor progress were normal. His parents became quite concerned about the CSF collection which had not disappeared by eight months, and he was referred back to the neurosurgeons. They found that the peritoneal catheter had blocked and it was therefore replaced.

After this, Michael began to get further problems and a series of four shunt revisions followed, each of which became infected. This culminated in the shunt's removal and the insertion of a ventricular drain. Michael had a respiratory arrest after one of the procedures and was comatose and in intensive care for several days. He made a full recovery from the respiratory arrest but required shunt revisions, all of which were unsuccessful because of infection. Eventually an external drainage system was inserted. Subsequently, attempts were made to clamp this off and treat the hydrocephalus with isosorbide, but this was not successful. A further ventriculo-peritoneal shunt was inserted, but this also became infected, and again external drainage was inserted. Michael's psychomotor development at about ten months of age had been a month or two behind, but then he contracted chickenpox from a ward visitor. This masked a further shunt infection, again with a rare organism, and status epilepticus developed. After failure of routine anticonvulsants to control this, he required intravenous thiopentone and remained in intensive care for several weeks.

When Michael recovered from this severe episode he had little or no visual or auditory attention, and spastic quadriplegia. There were also feeding difficulties suggesting severe bulbar problems.

Michael's parents were advised that it would be inappropriate to insert a ventriculo-peritoneal shunt until the CSF protein had fallen toward normal levels, and alternate-day CSF taps were performed on his Rickham reservoir. Michael made a little functional improvement after this, but a CT scan showed severe cerebral atrophy. It was felt that no more could be done in terms of neurosurgical intervention. The reservoir taps were continued after he was discharged home, and the CSF volumes decreased gradually. However, his head circumference continued to increase at a steady rate, and he developed severe hydrocephalus.

Michael's parents had lost all confidence in neurosurgical intervention, and we had great anxiety about the physical difficulties of managing a boy with gross hydrocephalus of a degree only seen in the era before the introduction of ventriculo-atrial shunts.

During this time Michael's parents had enrolled him on an intensive rehabilitation programme. In the course of three years they recruited a total of 150 volunteers, including some nurses and a physiotherapist from our department. They worked in shifts, usually of three people for one and a half to two hours twice a day carrying out passive exercises.

We felt that this was a very exacting programme for a boy with such severe disabilities, especially when his head size was increasing alarmingly. Nevertheless, we kept an open door for the family and put the parents in touch with various services, including the preschool adviser for visually impaired children and the occupational therapist from the social services department in case modifications were required to the home. His parents visited the nursery of the local special needs (severe) school and our team social worker was also involved.

When Michael and his parents came for follow-up appointments, consultation usually took place with my clinical assistant whose own daughter had been treated for hydrocephalus, and he was able to appreciate many of the anxieties which Michael's parents expressed. Although we did not approve of the intensity of the programme to which

Michael was being exposed, especially having seen a videotape of the exercises, we maintained contact with the family and our team helped with providing mobility aids and encouraging the setting up of a link family, and this was much appreciated by Michael's parents.

Michael's parents also tried acupuncture and acupressure for him. Eventually they were able to entrust his care to the local social services respite care team. This would have happened earlier but for the limited resources allocated to that area of care.

In his final illness, Michael's parents brought him to the children's ward. This they did on the advice of their general practitioner who had been a key figure of support and a major resource throughout Michael's short life.

Although medicine failed this family and they generated their own intervention programme, we felt it important to keep in touch and offer those services which were likely to be helpful, and to be taken up. It is very difficult with parents who are very keen to intervene, for those who are not involved operationally to say the programme is too intensive, or inappropriate, though there are occasions when we may need to do so even at the risk of losing the overall co-operation of the family and the ability to support them further when crises arise.

However, in this case there had been severe difficulties in managing a physical malformation, with catastrophic results. It is easy for doctors to identify with that failure and not to be positive, as the parents and their supporters were in this case, trying to do everything in their power to improve the outcome. Further, doctors are naturally more sceptical about unorthodox interventions than mainstream management, especially when orthodox treatment has failed.

A baby with psychomotor delay and visual problems following a neonatal illness
The uncertainty of outlook after a neonatal neurological illness can be difficult for both parents and paediatricians to cope with. Often an opinion from a paediatric neurologist at the tertiary referral centre will help direct investigations and give both the family and the local team confidence that the correct actions are being taken. If the neurologists work regularly with TDCs, their influence increases and so should their confidence in local service provision.

Joseph was the second child of healthy parents and the result of a normal pregnancy and delivery. He was born at 37 weeks gestation weighing 2950g. He was admitted to the ward at five days of age with marked jaundice. It was clear on first examination that he was an ill baby, with lethargy and pyrexia which had become gradually worse since birth. Initial investigation showed that he had mildly disordered clotting functions. Diagnoses of galactosaemia or disseminated intravascular coagulation were initially contemplated. Subsequent investigations for those conditions and a septic screen were negative. There was no evidence of intrauterine infection but his mother had been pyrexial with myalgia and a rash a week before he was delivered. Investigations in that direction, including viral studies, were also unrewarding. Joseph had been a breast-fed baby and had had only oral vitamin K at birth. It seemed quite possible that he had haemorrhagic disease of the new-born because his clotting corrected with intramuscular vitamin K. He developed transient myoclonic jerks and was hypotonic during this admission He was discharged at the age of 15 days.

Joseph was readmitted one week later with feeding problems and it was then noted that he was having having focal seizures; his electroencephalogram (EEG) showed multiple spike and wave activity, and at five weeks of age he was treated with phenobarbitone. He was seen by a paediatric neurologist because he had only fleeting eye fixation, poor eye contact and increased deep tendon jerks.

It was felt that he had evidence of an early motor disorder with hypotonia, increased reflexes and an abnormal EEG. His seizures and EEG pattern improved with prednisone therapy. His CT scan showed mild cerebral atrophy but his head circumference advanced normally.

Throughout Joseph's first year of life there were severe anxieties concerning his vision, to the extent that his parents even visited the local school for visually impaired children. He was enrolled on the Portage scheme (see Chapter 8) and made excellent progress. There were one or two setbacks and occasional seizures, but he continued to make steady progress. He was enrolled into the specialised day care nursery jointly funded by a local charitable organisation and the statutory bodies (education or social services depending on the child's special needs). His anticonvulsant treatment continued. He was referred to an ophthalmologist and was seen by the visiting teacher for visually impaired children. His parents obtained the statutory allowances for his disability and, through the local social services department, a link family was organised to help with his care and give the family some relief.

When he was three Joseph's vision was tested at 6/9 6/9 and N5 with his glasses. He had a residual squint and was still on anticonvulsants but his progress was excellent, and eventually at five years he was able to start in a mainstream school with one-to-one help from an extra teacher. Joseph's parents had their fourth child when he was four. During his preschool years Joseph's father was studying for and obtained a degree in educational psychology and his mother became one of the parent representatives on the management group of the TDC.

Again we have a family involved with many different agencies in the secondary and tertiary referral unit. There was a great deal of pressure on the mother of this family of four children, especially since the father was studying away from home for much of the time. Joseph was a child with a somewhat uncertain diagnosis and an equally uncertain prognosis, but eventually he was able to cope in mainstream schooling. His mother is now using her experiences to the benefit of others.

Sister with temporal lobe epilepsy and brother with Down syndrome
When there is more than one child in the family requiring significant medical input, it is better for the whole family to be looked after by the same team. The number of hospital attendances should be kept to a minimum by arranging simultaneous or consecutive clinic appointments for each child. This requires a flexible approach and care with organising appointments.

Cassie was first admitted to hospital at 22 months of age with a febrile convulsion. She had her third attack at 30 months and that lasted 15 minutes. During this time her mother was pregnant with her second child. Cassie was started on anticonvulsant therapy, developed normally, and had a normal EEG at four and a half years. Her therapy was discontinued at five and a half years.

Her first brother was born when she was two. Her second brother, Richard, was born four years later after a normal pregnancy and delivery. At two days he was noted to have the appearance of Down syndrome. Review of Richard's notes does not give an account of how the parents were told about his condition. They remember it as being unsatisfactory, with the mother alone being told first in the presence of students though both parents were told together later.

It was noted that there were no signs of congenital heart disease, and trisomy 21 was confirmed. Richard was quickly enrolled onto the Portage programme (Chapter 8) and his parents were referred for genetic counselling. Richard made good progress on Portage. He suffered a fractured tibia at the age of one year, and had an episode of altered consciousness at the age of two years. It was then noted on chest X-ray that he had a large heart. No murmur was heard but he had a loud pulmonary second sound and his electrocardiogram (ECG) showed right ventricular hypertrophy. He was referred for further investigation to the regional cardiac centre and was found to have primary pulmonary vascular disease. He required multiple admissions because of cardiac failure.

At about this time Cassie, who had previously had a total of five febrile convulsions, had a clonic/tonic attack lasting 10 minutes and her EEG showed a right temporal focus. Richard's cardiac condition continued to be somewhat precarious. He was enrolled into the day care nursery on a joint financing programme between a local charity and the education department. Several admissions to hospital ensued, often requiring urgent anti-failure treatment, including diamorphine.

The next year Cassie, now 11 years of age, had her second clonic/tonic attack, followed a year later by a further attack. She was started on long-term anticonvulsants which considerably improved her mood and there was no recurrence of attacks. She came off the anticonvulsants at 14 years of age.

In the meantime, Richard had developed *Pseudomonas aeruginosa* septicaemia and a urinary tract infection, and investigations showed a scar on his right kidney. Shortly after this he had a further admission with stridor due to acute epiglottitis. There were numerous other admissions and outpatient attendances. At the age of five years he started at his local special needs (severe) school.

Cassie, then 15 years old, had further seizures, and again a focus was seen on her EEG, while a CT scan showed mild atrophy of the contralateral temporal horn with a small CSF cyst and a small area of high enhancement which was thought not to be significant. Her anticonvulsants were restarted and she had no attacks in the following 11 months. At this time Richard was taken with the family on holidays abroad and was having fewer admissions, though undoubtedly the time will come when he will develop irreversible right ventricular failure. This family has coped extremely well with the double problem of having a boy with Down syndrome with a late diagnosis of primary pulmonary hypertension and a girl with moderately severe epilepsy.

Since Richard was born it has been our practice to perform ECGs and echo-cardiograms on all Down syndrome babies shortly after the birth, whether or not they have clinical signs of cardiac problems (Tubman *et al.* 1991).

It is also important to try to encourage families such as this to lead an ordinary family life, though this is difficult because many of their activities are centred on the hospital and on education for the special needs child. The mother of these children has since completed a counselling course and is offering her training and experience to help families with similar problems.

Sisters with 'cerebral palsy'
This family, initially with one able-bodied and one disabled girl, sought genetic advice through the TDC and the visiting neurologist and geneticist. Despite every effort to give the most informed advice possible, a second disabled child was born. The team continued to work with the family and communicate with all the other professionals from the tertiary referral centre, and the independent services that had been involved. The family has continued to use the services of the TDC despite their obvious misgivings concerning the genetic issue, and the lack of a definitive diagnosis.

Susan was brought by her parents for consultation at nine months of age because she was neither sitting unsupported nor babbling and her psychomotor development was clearly delayed.

She had been the result of a normal pregnancy and delivery, the second child of healthy non-consanguineous parents, and there were no neonatal problems to explain her psychomotor delay.

When first seen, Susan was very hypotonic but had preserved deep tendon reflexes. She sat supported with a very rounded back and had considerable head lag. She was felt to have global developmental delay and was referred to a paediatric neurologist. His view confirmed that the motor delay was explained by the severe hypotonia and that she was also intellectually behind. At 14 months of age her floppiness was resolving and she was developing increased motor tone with a symmetrical mixed motor problem worse in the legs than the arms. She was started on Portage (Chapter 8).

Though her parents were not planning further children at this stage, they were referred for genetic counselling. They were given an empirical risk of about one in eight of the situation recurring in subsequent children. Because this represented a high risk they were offered a CT brain scan for Susan to explore whether there was any structural brain abnormality which could indicate the origin of her problem and provide a better basis for estimating the risk of recurrence. This showed an abnormal density deep in the white matter, particularly adjacent to the lateral ventricles. These findings were discussed in detail by the geneticists, paediatric neurologists and the parents. The debates were protracted but the consensus emerged that the risk of recurrence was less than 10 per cent and that the abnormalities seen on scan probably represented the result of an acute intra-uterine event, unlikely to recur in subsequent pregnancies.

Susan's parents valued Portage as a local service delivered to their home, providing developmental advice on a specific basis, general support and contact with other local services and support groups. However, wanting to be sure that no possible remedies were left untried they also took Susan on a regular basis to a Spastics Society unit employing conductive education (see Chapter 8). This was about an hour's drive from their home and they visited once or twice a week. From this they were able to compare Susan's progress with similarly disabled children and explore a different style of intervention.

Like many parents of disabled children, Susan's sought opinions on her condition from other paediatric neurologists, and assessments by professionals working for The Spastics Society, but always with our knowledge.

A problem with single assessments performed by professionals working for voluntary or independent organisations is that by definition they only get a snapshot of the child. Rates of progress or evolution of events cannot be properly considered, and if a child is seen on a bad day the assessment may be invalid. Further, recommendations for intervention may well be made in ignorance of the level of service available locally to implement such recommendations. Nevertheless, assessments of this sort are often helpful in reassuring parents that the local services are appropriate and adequate.

In Susan's case, overall responsibility during this time always remained with our team, and the other opinions were supportive rather than confusing for her parents.

Susan had speech therapy to improve her language skills and oral motor control, and consideration was given to using augmentative communication methods and computers for the future. Susan's parents had a very busy time taking her to various local therapists and to consultations in regional centres.

When Susan was nearly five her mother became pregnant again; the pregnancy was monitored with high resolution ultrasound, and because of her age she had amniocentesis. Emily was the result of that normal pregnancy She was delivered normally and there were no difficulties with her in the neonatal period. However, at nine months she was brought for consultation and her problems were virtually identical to those with which Susan had presented at ten months. In fact, reading through Susan's notes after the consultation it was possible virtually to substitute one set of notes for the other. Our view at this point was that both children had an essentially ataxic/dystonic diplegia which had been inherited as an autosomal recessive disorder, and that the previous findings on the CT scan for Susan had been misleading. MRI was performed on Susan and there was a striking absence of myelin. Some form of leukodystrophy was suspected but further investigation failed to characterise it. Biopsies have been taken but so far no definite diagnosis has been made.

During this time both children had been attending the unit for conductive education on a regular basis. They also had physiotherapy, Portage and hydrotherapy. Susan is now attending a special school.

This is a family who have been at great pains to obtain genetic advice concerning the risks of having a second child with a problem. Despite their best efforts the problem did recur and they clearly carry an autosomal recessive gene for an as yet undefined neurological condition producing the manifestations of cerebral palsy.

A boy with spastic diplegia and girl with osteogenesis imperfecta
Families are dynamic and grow not only in numbers but also in their maturity and social

integration. TDCs too grow and evolve with members joining, growing with them and leaving. This is a family which 'grew up' in parallel with its local team, with mutual trust, cooperation and respect evolving as they grew.

Ashley was the first child of healthy parents. His mother was 24 years of age and she had been admitted to the antenatal ward for the last seven weeks of the pregnancy following an antepartum haemorrhage. She felt the pregnancy had reached 39 weeks but the baby's maturity was estimated as 35 weeks and he weighed 2520g. He was well at birth but was taken to the special care baby unit at six hours because of cyanosis. No intervention was required and he was discharged home at a few days of age. He was admitted overnight at three months of age when his mother had fallen downstairs with him.

At age 10 months Ashley was referred because of poor motor development. His GP requested a home visit and I saw him with his mother and health visitor. It was clear that he had an early mild spastic diplegia and a bilateral internal strabismus. The condition was explained to his mother and the management of physiotherapy and help with our domiciliary Portage scheme was offered and accepted. The health visitor stayed on after the consultation to make sure that Ashley's mother had understood the information which she had been given. Later that day she took a drug overdose but recovered quickly (I had overlooked the history of a previous overdose at 19 years of age).

Ashley made good progress on the Portage training scheme. Our medical social worker was closely involved with the family and there was good support from grandparents. Ashley's development was encouraging. When he was aged 13 months, his parents inquired about the risk for their second pregnancy and they were given the advice that as Ashley had been slightly preterm and there had been antepartum haemorrhage, it was relatively unlikely that a similar problem would occur in subsequent pregnancies.

When Ashley was 18 months of age, his mother gave birth to her second child. Melanie was born at 32 weeks gestation by breech delivery and weighed 1400g. She required ventilator therapy for two weeks because of congenital pneumonia. After Melanie's discharge home Ashley regressed in his feeding skills and suffered a febrile convulsion. In the first few weeks of Melanie's life the parents became rather despondent about Ashley's progress despite input from physiotherapy, Portage and hydrotherapy, and various other types of support.

At four months of age Melanie suffered a fracture of the right femur. The possibility of non-accidental injury was entertained, but it soon became apparent that she was suffering from osteogenesis imperfecta. Four months later that year she was admitted with hypothermia and cyanosis and a diagnosis of near-miss cot death was made. At about this time Ashley was starting at the day care nursery which specialises in special needs children. He also continued with Portage, and his Portage worker became the family key worker. It became apparent at this time that Melanie's psychomotor development was falling very much behind, but when appropriate help was given to the parents to work with Melanie her development accelerated dramatically. This suggested that most of the attention had previously been given to Ashley with the younger sister being rather marginalised. As more attention was given to Melanie and Portage was phased out for Ashley, he became somewhat jealous of the attention she was getting, but he made good progress and his development was normal at this stage, apart from his motor skills.

Melanie, when aged 10 months, suffered a further fracture when her mother was changing her nappy. At this time Melanie failed her hearing test, and at a chronological age of 12 months (nine months, corrected for gestational age), she was performing at a six month level. In the summer of that year Ashley had three febrile convulsions associated with otitis media and measles and in the autumn he underwent Achilles tendon lengthening procedures. This was followed up through our combined orthopaedic clinic. Both children were attending the local eye department for their squints and Melanie was having specialised otological consultations because of otosclerosis associated with osteogenesis imperfecta.

Because the family wanted to have more children they were referred to the regional genetics department and it was recommended that high resolution ultrasound screening of a subsequent pregnancy might give some reassurance. Subsequently the mother became pregnant again and her third child was delivered by caesarean section at 34 weeks because of premature rupture of membranes. The child was a healthy girl who remained completely well but she needed nursing in the special care baby unit for three weeks.

Adaptations to the home were organised by the social services occupational therapist. When he reached five years of age, Ashley started normal primary school. At this time Melanie was attending the specialised day nursery, and she joined Ashley in the mainstream school two years later. Both received extra help from welfare assistants. Because of problems with transport to school, negotiations with the education department led to rationalisation of their taxi journeys and modification of the teaching arrangements.

Through the next two years Ashley required further attention from the ear, nose and throat department because of drooling, and a referral to a regional orthopaedic surgeon for a baseline consideration of his diplegic gait. Ashley entered mainstream secondary school at 12 years. He has good mobility with elbow crutches, he touch types and he uses the computer keyboard.

Melanie is still well below the third centile for height and weight and at 11 years looks more like a six or seven year old. She has had numerous fractures, particularly in the legs, has radio hearing aids and still has amblyopia. She falls into the group of children with mild educational special needs, but she will always be vulnerable to fractures and uses a wheelchair.

This family has one child who is completely well and two with significant motor, physical and sensory problems. Over the years they have matured and grown in many respects and are now able to take initiatives in organising services for their children and utilise the voluntary and statutory services at their disposal in a constructive and rational way. They have come through very difficult times.

Ten years ago the father was living abroad and the family was considering emigrating. This was clearly unsettling for the family as a whole. They now are in control of their lives and are able to influence the social, educational, and health management of their children. This would not have been possible had the comprehensive umbrella of services organised through the TDC not been available to them and had it not encouraged their own self-sufficiency and independence.

A child with bizarre behaviours

A large proportion of children attending the TDC will have behavioural problems, which is a good reason for having easy access to psychology and psychiatry services. Sometimes, as in this case, the basis of the behavioural problem will be wrongly attributed and help from a tertiary specialist will be required. The specialist involved with the case described here is now conducting occasional clinics locally with our team to the benefit of both the team and the families involved.

Louise's mother had two grown-up children by her first marriage, and by her second marriage a daughter two years older and a son two years younger than Louise. She was aged 37 at Louise's birth and the father was 55. During the next few years the father developed an astrocytoma and required surgery, chemotherapy and radiotherapy. He suffered from convulsions and sudden severe mood changes. Louise was born normally at term but was small for gestational age at 2600g; the pregnancy had been complicated by ten days of vaginal bleeding at 28 weeks gestation. There were no neonatal problems and her parents first became worried at six months when they questioned her hearing.

She was referred to the CDC at three years by her GP. She had already been assessed by a community clinical medical officer (CMO) who had shown her to be functioning on the Griffiths Development Scale at between the 21 and 26 months level at 32 months of age. Her hearing and speech progress had been poor and grommets had been inserted for secretory otitis at one year. Subsequently at two and a half years audiometric assessment was normal. The CMO had already referred Louise for Portage which she started a month before her referral to the TDC; she had also been referred to the clinical psychologist working for the Community Learning Disability Team (CLDT).

When we first saw Louise, her parents' main concern was her disruptive behaviour and inability to appreciate danger. She was boisterous, spiteful and non-compliant. Her conduct was unpredictable; sometimes she was reasonable and lovable, sometimes she lapsed into prolonged bouts of screaming. She was of average stature and had an unusual facial appearance with mild ptosis and a 2cm depigmented area on the right flank. Her head circumference of 46.5cm was two two standard deviations below the mean. We did not feel that there was evidence of a neurocutaneous syndrome. Her chromosomes were normal and fragile X syndrome was ruled out—important because Louise's mother had two sisters each having a son with speech and language problems. Her outbursts could have been related to focal epilepsy, but her EEG was normal.

Despite intensive intervention from Portage and help from clinical psychologists and the CLDT nurse, Louise's behaviour became more bizarre and difficult. This included biting and kicking her brother, smearing faeces, spraying urine, eating from rubbish bins, and insomnia. Even with admission for five sessions per week to a special nursery and one week in six in residential care at a specialised unit, together with the previously mentioned interventions, the situation deteriorated.

We therefore made a referral to a developmental paediatrician and child psychiatrist at our regional centre. Louise and both parents attended with their key worker. Important observations were made at that consultation. These were that Louise's problems had begun at a very early age. She showed poor looking behaviours with avoidance of eye contact and she lacked reciprocal and social vocalisation. She threw toys rather than playing with them; she had hand regarding habits; and she did not gesture to be picked up though she did show attachment to her mother. By two years she would drag her mother's skirt to take her to what she wanted. Her mother would have to prepare a whole range of drinks from which Louise could select the one she wanted; if it was not available a tantrum would follow. Her symbolic play was virtually non-existent but she did communicate her needs for being picked up and cuddled. This was her main social contact; she did not share other social activities.

Louise seemed unaware of other people, unlike her younger brother who could 'suss out' situations, be aware of the feelings of others and modify his behaviour accordingly. Louise's tantrums would last for hours and they seemed to stem from anxiety and the fear of particular everyday objects and situations.

Given the developmental history and the signs and symptoms, a diagnosis of infantile autism was made. When this formulation was put to her parents it fitted well with their perceptions of the problem.

We had been put off this diagnosis by Louise's social approaching. This had misled us into misinterpreting her behaviours as resulting from frustration with her inability to communicate. The suggestion of temporal lobe attacks was in retrospect also unsupported.

From this consultation it emerged that the parents were already developing good strategies to cope with Louise's problems, but the TDC was able to give them a rather broader repertoire of interventions and explain the apparently irrational fears which were disturbing Louise. The team was also helpful in planning further educational placement and introducing the family to the National Autistic Society.

Children with autism are not common: in a population of about 50,000 under 16 years, we currently are involved with eight. Their presentation may not be typical, and as the spectrum of social–communication problems becomes more recognised, other children with less dramatic problems will come to light. The experience of specialists at a regional or tertiary referral level is invaluable in defining these children's problems and advising on management. A subgroup of our team is now taking a special interest in these very difficult children.

Quine and Pahl (1991) describe it as an important challenge to researchers to discover why some families cope in the face of severe stress, whilst others do not, and to understand what the elements of family functioning are which make some families vulnerable to stress and others able to resist it. They themselves found that being middle-class with few financial worries appears to buffer the effect of stressful behaviour for mothers of children with severe learning disability, showing the importance of utilitarian coping resources: such mothers can buy child-minding and cleaning services to give them a break from caring and household duties. They are also likely to be educated to a higher level, to have more access to information, and to have problem solving skills enabling them to formulate more positive coping strategies. They generally enjoy better health than working-class women. Mothers who had positive adjustment to, and acceptance of their children had lower stress scores. Mothers reporting little recent illness had higher health/energy/morale coping resources. Mothers feeling able to influence their own lives and achieve positive outcomes had lower scores on the malaise inventory.

There are therefore two main aspects to the TDC's work. The first involves the substrate—that is, the child–parent complex, their predicament, coping skills and health. This, as shown above, will determine the family's ability to survive stress. The other is represented by the resources co-ordinated, delivered or introduced by the TDC. The above findings may focus the team's attention on the families with fewer socioeconomic resources in order to promote and improve their coping abilities. Furthermore, Worley *et al.* (1991) have demonstrated in the USA that two financial counselling sessions supplemented by educational materials and telephone contact can lead to significant improvements in the financial management skills of parents of children with chronic disabilities.

REFERENCES

Cremers, M.J.G., Bol, E., de Roos, F., van Gijn, J. (1993) 'Risk of sports activities in children with Down's syndrome and atlantoaxial instability.' *Lancet*, **342**, 511–514.

Cunningham, C.C., Morgan, P.A., McGucken, R.B. (1984) 'Down's Syndrome : is dissatisfaction with disclosure of diagnosis inevitable?' *Developmental Medicine and Child Neurology*, **26**, 33–46.

Gage, J.R. (1992) *Gait Analysis in Cerebral Palsy. Clinics in Developmental Medicine No 121.* London: Mac Keith Press.

Gordon, N. (1993) 'Hereditary spastic paraplegia, a diagnostic reminder.' *Developmental Medicine and Child Neurology*, **35**, 452–455.

Hughes, I., Newton, R. (1992) 'Genetic aspects of cerebral palsy.' *Developmental Medicine and Child Neurology*, **34**, 80–86.

Quine, L., Pahl, J. (1987) 'First diagnosis of severe mental handicap: study of parental reactions.' *Developmental Medicine and Child Neurology*, **29**, 232–242.

—— —— (1991) 'Stress and coping in mothers caring for a child with severe learning difficulties: a test of Lazarus' transitional model of coping.' *Journal of Community and Applied Psychology*, **1**, 57–70.

Selby, K.A., Newton, R.W., Gupta, S., Hunt, L. (1991) 'Clinical predictors and radiological reliability in atlanto-axial subluxation in Down's syndrome.' *Archives of Disease in Childhood*, **66**, 876–878.

Selikowitz, M. (1993) 'A five year longitudinal study of thyroid function in children with Down syndrome.' *Developmental Medicine and Child Neurology*, **35**, 396–401.

Tubman, T.R.J., Shields, M.D., Craig, B.G., Mulholland, H.C., Nevin, N.C. (1991) 'Congenital heart disease in Down's syndrome: two year prospective early screening study.' *British Medical Journal*, **302**, 1425–1427.

Worley, G., Rosenfeld, L.R., Lipscomb, J. (1991) 'Financial counselling for families of children with chronic disabilities.' *Developmental Medicine and Child Neurology*, **33**, 679–689.

2
TERMINOLOGY IN DISABILITY

The World Health Organization (1980) has defined impairment, disability and handicap in terms of health experience, as set out below. It is recommended that these definitions be widely adopted; indeed, some editors insist on this (Jones 1987).

IMPAIRMENT

Definition

In the context of health experience, an impairment is any loss or abnormality of psychological, physiological, or anatomical structure or function
(Note : "Impairment" is more inclusive than "disorder" in that it covers losses – e.g., the loss of a leg is an impairment, but not a disorder)

Characteristics

Impairment is characterized by losses or abnormalities that may be temporary or permanent, and that include the existence or occurrence of an anomaly, defect, or loss in a limb, organ, tissue, or other structure of the body, including the systems of mental function. Impairment represents exteriorization of a pathological state, and in principle it reflects disturbances at the level of the organ

DISABILITY

Definition

In the context of health experience, a disability is any restriction or lack (resulting from an impairment) of ability to perform an activity in the manner or within the range considered normal for a human being

Characteristics

Disability is characterised by excesses or deficiencies of customarily expected activity performance and behaviour, and these may be temporary or permanent, reversible or irreversible, and progressive or regressive. Disabilities may arise as a direct consequence of impairment or as a response by the individual, particularly psychologically, to a physical, sensory, or other impairment. Disability represents objectification of an impairment, and as such reflects disturbances at the level of the person

Disability is concerned with abilities, in the form of composite activities and behaviours, that are generally accepted as essential components of everyday life. Examples include disturbances in behaving in an appropriate manner, in personal care (such as excretory control and the ability to wash and feed oneself), in the performance of other activities of daily living, and in locomotor activities (such as the ability to walk)

HANDICAP

Definition

In the context of health experience, a handicap is a disadvantage for a given individual, resulting from an impairment or a disability, that limits or prevents the fulfilment of a role that is normal (depending on age, sex, and social and cultural factors) for that individual

Characteristics	Handicap is concerned with the value attached to an individual's situation or experience when it departs from the norm. It is characterized by a discordance between the individual's performance or status and the expectations of the individual himself or of the particular group of which he is a member. Handicap thus represents socialization of an impairment or disability, and as such it reflects the consequences for the individual – cultural, social, economic, and environmental – that stem from the presence of impairment and disability
	Disadvantage arises from failure or inability to conform to the expectations or norms of the individual's universe. Handicap thus occurs when there is interference with the ability to sustain what might be designated as "survival roles"
Classification	It is important to recognize that the handicap classification is neither a taxonomy of disadvantage nor a classification of individuals. Rather is it a classification of circumstances in which disabled people are likely to find themselves, circumstances that place such individuals at a disadvantage relative to their peers when viewed from the norms of society

The key feature of the definition of handicap is that it is an outcome, not a cause. It may be the outcome of an impairment or a disability, but this is not exclusively the case. For example, a person may be handicapped because they perceive an impairment or disability which does not exist. Hence someone with an hysterical conversion syndrome may have the false perception of an impairment which leads to an experienced disability and consequent handicap. Conversely there are many mild impairments which do not necessarily lead to disability or handicap. More importantly and topically many individuals recognised as being disabled do not care to regard themselves as handicapped because they feel they can compete on their own terms with other members of society.

This is of course at odds with the WHO definition, for which the limitation or prevention of the fulfilment of a normal role indicates handicap. For example, as Pharoah (1990) reports:

One of the most moving personal accounts that distinguishes between disability and handicap was written by Stephen Hawking in his best selling book, *A Brief History of Time*. Motor neurone disease had confined Hawking to a wheelchair for over 20 years and the relentless progression of the disease had necessitated a tracheostomy which removed his ability to speak and made it almost impossible for him to communicate. It is difficult to imagine anyone having a more profound disability. Yet he goes on to say that he had led a fairly normal life having been fortunate to choose theoretical physics as a career, which is all in the mind, so that his disability was not a serious handicap!

It is also important to recognise that a single impairment may lead to a disability in a number of different spheres which are expressed as handicaps of different types: the impairments of cerebral palsy and spina bifida illustrate this well. In paediatrics, patients are not only the victims of their own impairments and disabilities but may also be the subject of other agents in their environment, particularly their parents or other carers. Environmental deprivation may result in a child becoming handicapped through neglect and lack of stimulation, and may compound the handicap of a child who is already disabled through other impairments. For example, the child who is hearing impaired and whose parents do not use the amplification system provided or recognise the need to use raised voice levels, may well be additionally handicapped as a result.

Notwithstanding the above we are often asked to deal with issues of physical handicap or learning disability on the assumption that they are completely separate entities. In some cases this approach is valid but someone who has a physical disadvantage might well be significantly affected by it both emotionally and socially. This may prejudice his or her learning opportunities resulting in a handicap in that area. Similarly, individuals with a significant burden of intellectual disability are seldom completely free of physical disadvantage. Again, using the model of spina bifida and hydrocephalus it can easily be shown how interdependent the physical and intellectual impairments and disabilities are and how the resulting handicap is a complex of numerous contributing factors.

The current interest in myalgic encephalomyelitis or postviral fatigue syndrome has served to polarise views of physical versus psychological illness. There are those who feel that the condition is entirely attributable to explicable physical agents and processes. Others feel that the apparent handicap of the sufferer is entirely psychologically determined, but most clinicians who have been involved in the management of patients who appear to have this condition would agree that the two mechanisms are not mutually exclusive and it is highly likely that both organic and psychological factors are involved (Gordon 1988, Walford *et al.* 1993). Unfortunately, in the area of childhood handicap, where physical and intellectual problems are often glaringly obvious, the emotional and psychological aspects, although present, are perhaps somewhat less obvious, and probably much more often overlooked than they are in a patient who starts from a more healthy baseline.

The WHO definition deals with handicap in the context of health experience, but for the purposes of the TDC, handicap has also to be explored in its social and educational contexts. There is no question that the child's environment has a major influence on allowing or disallowing the achievement of his or her potential: thus the whole social background including all aspects of nurturing, such as housing, clothing and nutrition, must be considered along with tenderness, identity, discipline and other parenting characteristics which carers may or may not provide.

The major difference between the speciality of paediatrics and general medicine is that the healthy child grows and develops in all areas of ability and represents a much more dynamic entity than the adult. The child with a disability, however, will often grow and develop at a different rate from those in the normal population. For example, children with Sotos syndrome who grow at a very rapid rate during the first few years of life may be perceived as older than they are, but this becomes a double handicap when their intellectual capacity is below chronological age: a six-year-old looking eight years old and behaving as a four-year-old. Similarly, a very bright child with short stature, for whatever reason, may be treated as a five-year-old when s/he is in fact seven years of age but should be treated intellectually as an eight- or nine-year-old. Growth impairment may cause a disability inasmuch as the child is unable to see over obstructions as well as friends can, but the major handicap comes from being inappropriately treated as a younger child than s/he is, and as a much younger child than his or her intellectual ability deserves.

Children with dynamic problems such as the progressive degenerative disorders have changing needs requiring different kinds of management as they grow older. For instance, children with Batten's disease require change in schooling and general management because of failing visual competence, introduction of anticonvulsants for seizures and finally progressively more care because of greater dependency as intellectual and physical abilities are lost. Also, children with non-progressive impairments—cerebral palsy, for example—have changing needs as they grow older because the manifestations of the condition change with the maturation of the central nervous system and the musculo-skeletal system, and with physical growth.

For these reasons it is very difficult to give prescriptions for management of children with a particular kind of disability. Only generalisations can be made and certain features highlighted by case descriptions. We need to evaluate all the influences which may be acting on the child at any one time, including those deriving from the disease, age and environment complex of the patient.

Screening, surveillance and assessment

The basic terminology has been changed and perhaps devalued over time. Whitmore and Bax (1988) consider that neither 'screening' nor 'surveillance' are semantically correct terms for the work of health examinations. Both they and Stone (1990) quote Wilson and Jungner (1968) as authorities on screening, together with the Commission on Chronic Illness (1957), and the criteria quoted by Cochrane and Holland (1971) may be added to those texts. Using strict criteria, Whitmore and Bax conclude that examination and assessment are the key processes in checking the health of an individual and they are carried out by skilled professionals, whereas screening a given population for a particular condition is usually carried out by less skilled personnel. Screening is certainly a valid term when used to describe blood testing on all neonates for phenylketonuria or congenital hypothyroidism, but few other procedures in child health qualify under this term.

Whitmore and Bax advise that parents whose children are late in sitting, walking or talking, or who are clumsy or have visual and hearing defects or behavioural problems (such as sleep disturbance, temper tantrums or learning difficulties) need immediate help with these problems, just as they do for a child with an infection. There is abundant evidence that such problems are common and that many children who have them fare less well in later life. Therefore it is crucial that they receive early attention. For many of these problems, there are no valid screening tests that can be easily and readily applied, and parents do not always realise that their child may have a problem for which help should be obtained.

In contrast, child health doctors and nurses through their regular examinations and parental interviews can readily identify not only abnormal physical conditions, but also developmental and behavioural disorders. It may be argued that there are no clear-cut ways of managing the latter, but for centuries doctors have seen it as a duty to try to help patients with disorders which are not yet fully understood and whose remedy therefore is difficult.

Hall and colleagues (1989) suggested a new programme for child health surveillance.

This was criticised by Bax and Whitmore (1990) for having 'a terrible muddle about screening, examinations and surveillance'. Wilson (1990) acknowledged that Hall's section on screening for developmental impairments had caused controversy among professionals but agreed that detailed developmental screening is unnecessary. But in fact Hall and colleagues are not screening in the true sense: they are systematically examining whole populations in the style suggested by Bax and Whitmore. Colver (1990), while applauding the publication by Hall and colleagues, came to a final rational conclusion that 'in the present state of knowledge the emphasis should rightly be shifted from repeated detailed examinations of children who happen to come to a clinic to the systematic examination of all children using a small number of tests uniformly applied.' This is certainly at odds with Hall's recommendations and leaves the small number of tests and their validation to be defined.

In 1990 Stone tried to clarify the position. In addition to the problems with definition of handicap, he outlined other problems with terminology in community child health and proposed definitions of surveillance, monitoring, screening, assessment and examination. His definitions and comments are reproduced in full below:

SURVEILLANCE

Child health surveillance is the systematic and ongoing collection, analysis, and interpretation of indices of child health, growth, and development in order to identify, investigate and, where appropriate, correct deviations from predetermined norms.

Surveillance may be of two kinds: *clinical surveillance*, which focuses on the individual child, and *population surveillance*, in which data are recorded on a group, community, or entire population of children. Clinical surveillance enables an early clinical diagnosis to be reached when an abnormality is identified, regardless of whether or not the abnormality is treatable, while population surveillance provides the database for the early formulation of a community diagnosis.

Comment

The definition proposed here is comparable with that which is widely used in the public health literature and is usually synonymous with monitoring. It implies data collection and analysis at a population level with a view to detecting deviations from a predetermined norm. (Preventative and other interventions, such as immunisation, may be initiated by surveillance but are not an intrinsic part of it.) The main purpose of surveillance is the gathering of information for facilitating the reaching of a diagnosis. The routine measurement and recording of height, weight, and developmental progress of individual children is therefore a form of clinical surveillance, as the discovery of deviations from population norms is the *raison d'etre* of this type of activity. Aggregated growth and development data from a large number of children may be analysed to monitor the health of a total population. While it is useful to distinguish between clinical and population surveillance, in practice the database for both is generated in an identical manner.

MONITORING

Monitoring is synonymous with surveillance (see above).

SCREENING

Screening is not intended to be diagnostic, but is the presumptive identification of unrecognised disease or defects by the application of tests, examinations, and other procedures designed to facilitate early diagnosis followed by prompt and effective treatment.

Comment

Unlike surveillance, which means intelligence gathering, screening is intended to initiate a chain of events, including diagnosis and treatment, which ultimately benefit the individual by halting or reversing the natural history of a disease process. Screening is therefore a form of clinical prevention. Criteria have been established to assist planners assess whether or not a screening test is worthwhile. It is most effective when aimed at the detection and treatment of specific, treatable abnormalities such as visual and hearing defects in young children or hypothyroidism in neonates. As the use of periodic examination to monitor growth and development is a form of surveillance rather than an explicitly preventive activity, the term 'developmental screening' is a misnomer. The application of screening criteria to surveillance is consequently inappropriate.

ASSESSMENT

Assessment is the systematic, detailed, and multidisciplinary examination of the physical, emotional, and social health of a child with suspected or established disability or disadvantage.

Comment

The aim of an assessment is to reach an appropriate series of clinical decisions for the child with special needs. It is usually undertaken in assessment centres, and is relevant only to the minority of children with disabilities. This minority should be identifiable in the course of surveillance. The term should not be used interchangeably with surveillance, screening, or examination, all of which are applicable to all children in the community.

EXAMINATION

Examination is the action of establishing the clinical state of a child by means of a combination of questioning, testing, and observing the child in the context of a professional relationship.

Comment

Examination is a generic term used to denote any fact finding activity, though it is usually clinical in nature. It conveys no implicit or explicit purpose, which may be diagnostic, preventive, therapeutic, or administrative. Consequently, it serves no useful function other than as a description of data collection undertaken by a professional.

In conclusion, Stone states that we need to reach a consensus in these issues, saying that without a wide measure of agreement on basic terminology, fruitful discussion of the underlying concepts is impossible.

REFERENCES

Bax, M.C.O., Whitmore, K. (1990) 'Health for all children.' *Archives of Disease in Childhood*, **65**, 141–142.

Cochrane, A.L., Holland, W.W. (1971) 'Validation of screening procedures.' *British Medical Bulletin*, **27**, 3–8.

Colver, A. (1990) 'Health for all children.' *Archives of Disease in Childhood*, **65**, 142. *(Letter.)*

Commission on Chronic Illness (1957) *Chronic Illness in the United States, Vol. 8. Prevention of Chronic Illness.* Cambridge, MA: Harvard University Press.

Gordon, N. (1988) 'Myalgic encephalomyelitis.' *Developmental Medicine and Child Neurology*, **30**, 677–682.

Hall, D.M.B. (Ed.) (1989) *Health for All Children: A Programme for Child Health Surveillance. The Report of the Joint Working Party on Child Health Surveillance.* Oxford: Oxford University Press.

Hawking, S.W. (1988) *A Brief History of Time.* London: Bantam Press.

Jones, B. (1987) 'Impairment, disability and handicap.' *Child: Care, Health and Development*, **13**, 359. *(Editorial.)*

Pharoah, P.O.D. (1990) 'Impairment, disability, and handicap.' *Archives of Disease in Childhood*, **65**, 819. *(Annotation.)*

Stone, D.H. (1990) 'Terminology in community child health—an urgent need for consensus.' *Archives of Disease in Childhood*, **65**, 817–818. *(Annotation.)*

Walford, G.A., Nelson, W. McC., McCluskey, D.R. (1993) 'Fatigue, depression, and social adjustment in chronic fatigue syndrome.' *Archives of Disease in Childhood*, **68**, 384–388.

Whitmore, K., Bax, M.C.O. (1988) 'Screening or examining?' *Developmental Medicine and Child Neurology*, **30**, 673–676.

Wilson, J.A. (1990) 'Health for all children.' *Archives of Disease in Childhood*, **65**, 142. *(Letter.)*

Wilson, J.M.G., Jungner, G. (1968) *Principles and Practise of Screening for Disease. WHO Public Health Papers No 34*. Geneva: WHO.

World Health Organization (1980) *International Classification of Impairments, Disabilities and Handicaps. A Manual of Classification Relating to the Consequences of Disease*. Geneva: WHO.

3
THE AVERAGE HEALTH DISTRICT

In the UK there are 17 (soon to be reduced to eight) Regional Health Authorities divided into 192 District Health Authorities (many now becoming National Health Service Trusts). A Health District on average has an adult population of about 250,000 and a childhood population under 15 years of around 40,000–60,000. This is comparable to a county in Denmark but smaller than the 365,000 overall population of an average county in Sweden. At present most District Health Authorities would be served by two or three general paediatricians and one or two consultant paediatricians in community child health who are gradually replacing principal medical officers in child health. The tertiary paediatric specialists, such as consultant paediatric neurologists and neurodevelopmental paediatricians, are based in the regional centres but may conduct clinics in the district hospitals and especially in the CDCs. Referrals to them are mainly by general paediatricians or consultant paediatricians in community child health, and patients who are referred by their GPs are usually seen by consultant paediatricians.

The prevalence of cerebral palsy in the UK is about two per 1000, and that of both Down syndrome and neural tube defects (spina bifida and hydrocephalus) about one per 1000. This is put in perspective by the fact that, while overall 20 per cent of the school population will have special educational needs at some time with as many as 17 per cent at any one time (Warnock 1978), only one tenth of those children will actually receive education in special schools. It has been estimated that half of them will require regular contact with the DHT or TDC (Neville 1986). This means that in the average Health District there will be about 500 children who require regular contact of some form with the TDC.

Similarly, in Ontario Cadman et al. (1986), using parental questionnaire responses concerning 3294 children (age range 4–16 years) selected by stratified, clustered random sampling from the 1981 census population, found that 19.6 per cent of these children had some form of chronic health problem (Tables 3.1–3.4). This very large prevalence included 14 per cent with chronic illness without functional limitations, 1.9 per cent with limitations of function not associated with chronic illness, and 3.7 per cent with a chronic illness or medical condition accompanied by limitation of function. They also found an association between chronic health problems and poverty.

The Office of Population Censuses and Surveys (OPCS) Report No. 3 on Disability in Great Britain (Bone and Meltzer 1989) gives details of types of disability and severity as calculated from parental questionnaires (Table 3.5). Behavioural problems represent the largest disability group in this study.

Köhler and Jakobsson (1987) in their book *Children's Health and Well-being in the Nordic Countries* devoted a chapter to chronically ill and handicapped children. They pointed out that 'no one really knows how many chronically ill and handicapped children

TABLE 3.1

**Limitations of normal function in 157 children in the
Ontario Child Health Study***

Limitation	N
Physical activity	
Limited in the kind or amount of vigorous activity	83
Trouble walking several blocks or climbing few flights of stairs	29
Trouble bending, lifting or stooping	14
Unable to walk without assistance	1
Mobility	
Needs help or supervision in using transportation	12
Needs help or supervision in getting around neighbourhood	15
Self-care	
Needs help with eating, dressing, bathing or using toilet	10
Role	
Limited in kind or amount of ordinary play	51
Limited in kind or amount of schoolwork	73
Unable to attend school	12

*Age range 4–16 years. Weighted prevalence of at least one
limitation = 56/1000.
Reproduced by permission from Cadman *et al.* (1986).

there are in the Nordic countries (or in any other country for that matter)', adding that published data are unreliable because the reasons for collection vary widely, the studies are of a variety of populations in a variety of geographic areas; and the methods of data collection are not standard. Of particular importance is the reason for data collecting: those with a special interest or wanting to generate support for research may tend to exaggerate the numbers, while those responsible for providing welfare funding and looking for savings may have a higher diagnostic threshold.

Köhler and Jakobsson quoted overall prevalence rates for chronic disease among children aged two to 18 years of 6.3 per cent (Denmark), 9.8 per cent (Finland), 9.6 per cent (Norway) and 7.5 per cent (Sweden). Data are broken down by age-groups in Table 3.6 (Finland), Table 3.7 (Norway) and Table 3.8 (Sweden).

Comparing these figures with the UK OPCS data the major difference is in the reporting of disability related to behaviour. This is almost certainly a result of differences in methods of data collection and analysis, the Nordic surveys looking at disease, and the OPCS at disability.

Köhler and Jakobsson concluded by stating:

It is very difficult to get a complete picture of the occurrence of chronic illness in children in the Nordic countries. The only unanimous information concerns disease groups, *e.g.* that the children's

TABLE 3.2

**Chronic illnesses or medical conditions in 528 children
in the Ontario Child Health Study***

Illness/condition	N
Total blindness in one or both eyes†	10
Vision problem even with glasses†	26
Deafness†	14
Hearing problem but not deafness†	33
No speech†	7
Speech problems†	95
Moderate or severe pain†	83
Asthma	94
Heart problem	55
Epilepsy or convulsions without fever	23
Kidney disease	9
Arthritis or rheumatism	25
Cerebral palsy	3
Muscular dystrophy or muscle disease	2
Spina bifida	1
Diabetes	3
Cancer	2
Cystic fibrosis	2
Missing limb(s)	3
Physical deformity	74
Paralysis or weakness of any kind	12
Other chronic health problem	135

*Age range 4–16 years. Weighted prevalence of at least one
chronic illness or medical condition = 177/1000.
†Of at least 6 months duration.
Reproduced by permission from Cadman *et al.* (1986).

chronic diseases are mostly found in the groups: sensory organs, respiratory system and diseases affecting the skin and subcutaneous tissues. Of the 'classic' handicaps, mental retardation is most common (about eight per 1000), epilepsy and heart defects (about four per 1000), and cerebral palsy, hydrocephalus, diabetes (between one and two per 1000). A considerable fraction are multi-handicapped. Information on the total occurrence of chronic illness varies from 1.5 per cent to 16 per cent of all children. The variation is at least partly dependent on the definition of chronic illness and the survey procedure. It may be said that the proportion of chronically ill children decreases the stricter the medical definition and the more precise the survey methods used. The interview method, which has a vaguer definition of chronic illness, has the advantage that it gives information on how chronic illness is distributed. The surveys referred to state that 7 to 19 per cent of children have some form of chronic illness. Chronic illness is nearly without exception more common among boys than among girls. Evidence indicates that chronic illness increases with age, but the results are equivocal. The association between social group and chronic illness is very unclear. On the one hand it may be shown that there is no association whatsoever, and on the other hand chronic illness is more common partly in high status groups and partly in low status groups. The same applies to the regional distribution of chronic illness. In some surveys no differences have been found, and in others the differences have been great.

TABLE 3.3

Weighted prevalence rates of chronic health problems per 1000 children, by age and sex, in the Ontario Child Health Study

Health problem	Boys		Girls		Total (and 95% confidence interval
	4–11 yrs	12–16 yrs	4–11 yrs	12–16 yrs	
Limitation of normal function alone	18	27	8	28	19 (13–25)
Chronic illness or condition alone	163	146	115	138	140 (125–155)
Chronic illness or condition and limitation of normal function	29	58	18	52	37 (29–45)
Total	210	231	141	218	196 (179–213)

Reproduced by permission from Cadman *et al.* (1986).

TABLE 3.4

Weighted prevalence rates of chronic health problems per 1000 children, by socioeconomic status, in the Ontario Child Health Study

Health problem	Below poverty line	Above poverty line
Limitation of normal function alone	31	16
Chronic illness or condition alone	160	133
Chronic illness or condition and limitation of normal function	46	34
Total	237	183

Reproduced by permission from Cadman *et al.* (1986).

TABLE 3.5

Estimates of prevalence of disability among children in Great Britain by type of disability and age (rate per 1000 population)

Type of disability	0–4 yrs	5–9 yrs	10–15 yrs
Locomotion	5	10	11
Reaching and stretching	2	2	2
Dexterity	2	4	4
Seeing	2	2	2
Hearing	3	8	6
Personal care	6	10	7
Continence	6	14	8
Communication	5	13	13
Behaviour	13	23	25
Intellectual functioning	4	9	12
Consciousness	5	5	5
Eating, drinking, digestion	1	1	0
Disfigurement	1	1	2

Adapted by permission from Bone and Meltzer (1989).

33

TABLE 3.6

Chronic illness in children in Finland 1976 according to disease group, age and sex (%)

Disease groups	0–6 yrs		7–14 yrs		0–14 yrs	
	Boys	Girls	Boys	Girls	Boys	Girls
Nervous and sensory organs	20.4	21.2	28.0	26.5	25.9	25.1
Respiratory system	14.8	13.6	11.9	24.3	12.7	21.4
Skin and subcutaneous tissues	7.4	19.7	13.3	11.3	11.7	13.6
Uro-genital organs	20.4	3.0	14.0	2.3	15.7	2.5
Musculo-skeletal	9.3	7.6	6.3	6.2	7.1	6.6
Mental illness	5.6	6.1	3.5	6.8	4.1	6.5
Others	22.2	28.8	23.1	22.6	22.8	24.3

Köhler and Jakobsson (1987).

TABLE 3.7

Chronic illness in children in Norway 1975, according to disease groups, age and sex (rate per 1000 children)

Disease groups	0–6 yrs		7–15 yrs	
	Boys	Girls	Boys	Girls
All disease groups	131.8	121.9	223.7	173.3
Nervous disorders and symptoms	4.9	3.8	12.4	10.9
Diseases of the nervous system	3.3	—	2.3	6.1
Diseases of the eyes and ears	11.5	5.7	22.6	17.0
Coronary and vascular disease	1.6	—	1.1	—
Diseases of the respiratory system	36.3	38.1	61.0	27.9
Gastric ulcer, catarrh and other gastric conditions	—	—	—	1.2
Other diseases of the digestive tract	3.3	1.9	3.4	3.6
Diseases of the uro-genital organs	3.3	15.3	3.4	18.2
Diseases of the skin and subcutaneous tissues	47.8	38.1	61.0	53.3
Musculo-skeletal diseases	9.9	3.8	27.1	19.4
Other diseases	6.6	11.4	18.1	12.1
Injuries	3.3	3.8	11.3	3.6

Köhler and Jakobsson (1987).

The epidemiology of cerebral palsy has engaged many devoted workers in a search for causative factors (Stanley and Alberman 1984). Hagberg *et al.* (1989) produced data detailing the changing and subsequent stabilisation of incidence and prevalence of various types of cerebral palsy in Sweden. More recently, Mutch *et al.* (1992) outlined the current difficulties of case definition, comparability of cases, impairments, disability levels and their description. One of the most researched areas of childhood disability remains one of the most difficult to classify both in terms of clinical features and of aetiology.

Although when they did their survey in 1985 Bax and Whitmore found that some DHTs were seeing children with asthma, cystic fibrosis and congenital heart disease, most teams would feel that the children with those conditions are best dealt with in the general acute paediatric outpatient clinic or in joint consultation with regional specialists (tertiary referral), especially in the case of cystic fibrosis or congenital heart disease. Of course some

34

TABLE 3.8

Numbers of children and adolescents with paediatric disease or disability in Sweden 1983 (from a total population of 2,139,452 in the age group 0–19 years)

Disease/disability	Prevalence per 1000	N (all)	N (severely disabled)
Neurological disease			
Cerebral palsy	1.7	3800	1000
Spina bifida	0.45[1]	1000	650
Muscular disease	0.25–0.35	600–800	400
Epilepsy (attack during last 3 years)	4	8900	2000
Hydrocephalus	1.1 (4–7 yrs)	2000	2000
Minimal brain dysfunction	40–71 (6–10 yrs) Severe 12	?	27,000
Other paediatric diseases			
Asthma	15	33,300	1000
Severe skin diseases	?	?	?
Haemophilia	0.14	300	100
Cystic fibrosis	0.09	200	200
Diabetes	1.3 (0–14 yrs)	2900	100
Heart defects	0.3	650	650
Chronic juvenile (rheumatoid) arthritis	0.6 (school age)	1300	400
Tumours		About 275 new cases per year	
Others			
Mental retardation	8	17,800	7500
Severe	3	6700	6700
Slight and moderate	5	11,100	2000[2]
Visual defects	1.5–2	3300–4400	2000–2600
Serious visual defects	0.4	900	900
Deaf and blind	0.04	80	80
Hearing defects	1.8	4000	1400
Deafness	0.6	1300	1300
Language and speech defects	?	?	?
Child psychosis	0.5	1100	1100
Malformations of extremities	0.45	1000	?
Cleft lip and palate	1.4	3100	?
Ileo-, colo- and urostomy operations	0.1	250	250
Locomotor ataxia total	4.1	9100	3300

[1]0.60 at birth.
[2]First and foremost dependent on multiple disability.
Adapted from Köhler and Jakobsson (1987).

of the cases which were reported to Bax and Whitmore would have been children who had these conditions in addition to the more usual problems dealt with by the DHT, such as complicated Down syndrome. In order to make the most efficient use of resources, especially where children are being seen by a team in a simultaneous consultation, it is not appropriate to see children with conditions which could equally well or better be dealt with in an ordinary consultation with the paediatrician or another member of the team. For example, half the children with cerebral palsy will have hemiplegia. For many of them this will be so mild that they do not need to attend a consultation with the full team on a regular basis, and follow-up by the paediatrician with the physiotherapist is usually adequate for that group of children, with perhaps occasional joint consultations with an orthopaedic surgeon. Similarly, whether a child with epilepsy is dealt with on a regular basis by the TDC will depend to a large extent on the other problems, such as intellectual disability, cerebral palsy or any other underlying primary neurological syndrome, rather than just the epilepsy. In practice, most of the children with epilepsy will be dealt with in the general paediatric clinic.

Another particularly difficult area is the child with developmental delay of uncertain aetiology. Whilst it is important that the child is investigated in order to establish aetiology and identify the extent of the intellectual problems, once this has been done it is not reasonable to bring the child back, especially after school entry age, to a multidisciplinary clinic when the problem remains mainly one of educational difficulties.

Should all children with psychomotor problems be registered with the TDC? It would certainly be easier for the TDC professionals in the UK to fulfil their obligations to the Social Services Department if this were the case. In the UK, the Children Act (1989) obliges professionals to notify Social Services of children with special (educational or other) needs. Thus if every child with special needs, or with the potential for having special needs, were registered with the TDC when first seen, this obligation would be more easily fulfilled. On the other hand, the special needs of the child might have resolved by the time school age is reached and then deregistration would be required. Nevertheless, for the TDC properly to plan its services in the light of the needs of the local population, an early registration system should be encouraged.

The more difficult area is where the paediatrician in the TDC is not aware of all the special needs children being seen by his or her other paediatric colleagues who for various reasons have not referred them to the TDC. Often TDC statistics will underestimate the number of children with special needs within a health authority because some children are being followed up by a paediatrician in a different clinic who either does not know about the service available from the TDC or is reluctant to refer on some other grounds. Sometimes paediatricians have difficulty in disengaging from families whom they have helped through stormy episodes, while families often feel reluctant to let go or change their professional advisors. In such cases, what should be remembered is that referral to the TDC has the advantage of a built-in second opinion.

As a minimum, it does seem rational that there should be a system run by the TDC for registering all special needs children attending hospital clinics, which means that data concerning children who attend general or specialised clinics other than the TDC, but who will require the services of the TDC, would be fed into the system (see Chapter 10). This might trigger the implementation of needed but as yet unprovided services for those children.

In some health authorities there will be a register of special needs children with data shared between the TDC and the community child health service or even a common information system, and often, of course, the TDC is organised and led by the community service.

If the above systems can be activated it is much easier for school medical officers and doctors working in community clinics to be in full possession of relevant data for these children and to provide a more efficient surveillance service for school and preschool children.

REFERENCES

Bax, M.C.O., Whitmore, K. (1985) *District Handicap Teams: Structure, Function and Relationships. Report to DHSS.* London: Community Paediatric Research Unit, Westminster Children's Hospital.

Bone, M., Meltzer, H. (1989) *The Prevalence of Disability among Children. OPCS Surveys of Disability in Great Britain. Report 3.* London: HMSO.

Cadman, D., Boyle, M., Offord, D.R., Szatmari, P., Rae-Grant, N.I., Crawford, J., Byles, J. (1986) 'Chronic illness and functional limitations in Ontario's children: findings of the Ontario Child Health Study.' *Canadian Medical Association Journal*, **135**, 761–767.

Hagberg, B., Hagberg, G., Zetterstrom, R. (1989) 'Decreasing perinatal mortality: increase in cerebral palsy morbidity.' *Acta Paediatrica Scandinavica*, **78**, 664-670.

Köhler, L., Jakobsson, G. (1987) *Children's Health and Well-being in the Nordic Countries. Clinics in Developmental Medicine No. 98.* London: Mac Keith Press.

Mutch, L., Alberman, E., Hagberg, B., Kodama, K., Perat, M.V. (1992) 'Cerebral palsy epidemiology: where are we now and where are we going?' *Developmental Medicine and Child Neurology*, **34**, 547–551.

Neville, B.G.R. (1986) *Services for Chronic Disability in Childhood and Adolescence in the United Kingdom. BPA/BPNA Working Party Report to the DHSS.*

Stanley, F., Alberman, E. (Eds.) (1984) *The Epidemiology of the Cerebral Palsies. Clinics in Developmental Medicine No. 87.* London: S.I.M.P.

Warnock Report (1978) *Special Educational Needs. Report of the Committee of Enquiry into the Education of Handicapped Children and Adults. Cmnd 7212.* London: HMSO.

4
THE MULTIDISCIPLINARY TEAM

Service models for the multidisciplinary TDCs can take several forms. Their structure, manning levels and management will depend on which service model is adopted. Bax and Whitmore (1991), in their review of 'District Handicap Teams' (DHTs) in England 1983–88, analysed on two separate occasions the composition and activities of such teams and found surprising heterogeneity in both membership and scope of activities. They pointed out that by 1988 only 37 per cent of health districts had what they regarded as a DHT as defined by the Court Committee (1976). They went on to make recommendations based on the Child Development Centre (CDC), outlining the range of professionals who should be involved with its function but carefully avoiding the issue of the operational functions of the DHT. The recommendations are important and are reproduced in Chapter 5. The probable reason why only a minority of health districts in England had developed DHTs by 1988 is that the key individuals, namely hospital- or community-based consultant paediatricians, had not had the appropriate training and experience of working in teams. As that experience becomes more widespread and accepted as normal, the number of properly constituted DHTs or TDCs ought to increase.

Service models
Rosenbloom (1985) identified three types of clinical service models which in various ways provide and integrate clinical services for children with disabilities. These are (i) multidisciplinary assessment (evaluation), (ii) comprehensive care, and (iii) registration and monitoring.

The pattern of professional involvement for each of these models would be determined by the type and pattern of service offered.

Multidisciplinary assessment
Two basic patterns of assessment services are commonly seen. The first of these is 'Do it all', which is sequential multidisciplinary assessment in which referred children go through all aspects of a predetermined assessment procedure. Commonly in this type there is a preliminary introduction and explanation by a social worker or health visitor; then in turn there are medical examinations including assessments of vision and hearing, educational or psychological assessments, and various therapy assessments; then there is usually a conference with or without the parents, following which a report is made to the referring authority and often in current practice to the parents also.

This type of assessment is time consuming and can usually only be offered to selected children within a particular community, *e.g.* the most severely disabled.

There has been a tendency for this type of assessment to take place at tertiary referral units rather than at the district level. It has to be carefully planned and executed, and is expensive, labour intensive and extremely demanding on the child and parents, especially if the whole exercise is completed in one day rather than in sessions spread over a series of days.

The second type of multidisciplinary assessment that Rosenbloom identified was 'Selective assessment'. Here, the service in the CDC acts as a supplement to other services. For example, the community child health service may have carried out a developmental assessment. The function of the disabled children's service is to identify any gaps in the assessment, and review and perhaps provide therapy for individual children. It needs adequate resources available to fill these gaps. In such a service, more disabled children can be seen than in the first model, and good use can be made of resources that might be scarce in any particular service or community. Such a pattern can avoid duplication of use of resources, but does demand effective co-ordination.

Comprehensive care
The multidisciplinary team will not only undertake assessment and evaluation of the needs of the child and family but ought to be able to provide within the local services the facilities and personnel for continuous support therapies and reassessment. To quote Rosenbloom, 'Such a system implies that there will be a single co-ordinated service for disabled children in the particular community. There will be appropriate selection of the professionals who will need to see those children and their families.' Often the nomination of key workers will promote this activity.

Registration and monitoring
Some teams function only as data collection bases for organising the registration of children with special educational needs, and collecting data for planning a clinical service and future functions. Bax and Whitmore (1985) found within this subheading some DHTs who did very little clinical evaluation or intervention, and whose main function was organising case conferences, collating information from different agencies, and making recommendations on the basis of those data. This does not fulfil the functional role of the teams where the day-to-day clinical management of the child and family is one of the fundamental activities.

Usual styles
Most teams function on the basis of being able to arrange comprehensive assessment. This does not necessarily take place in a sequential manner on one day, in one place, but may be gathered together over a period of time using information from members of the team and other competent professionals in whom the team has confidence. This information is then collated and recommendations are made for the care plan for the child.

Some teams function on a core basis, having only three to six professionals as members of the core group. This provides paediatric, social work, therapeutic, psychological and educational input, and the consultations take place on a joint basis with appropriate members of the core team present. When other assessments are required, referrals are made

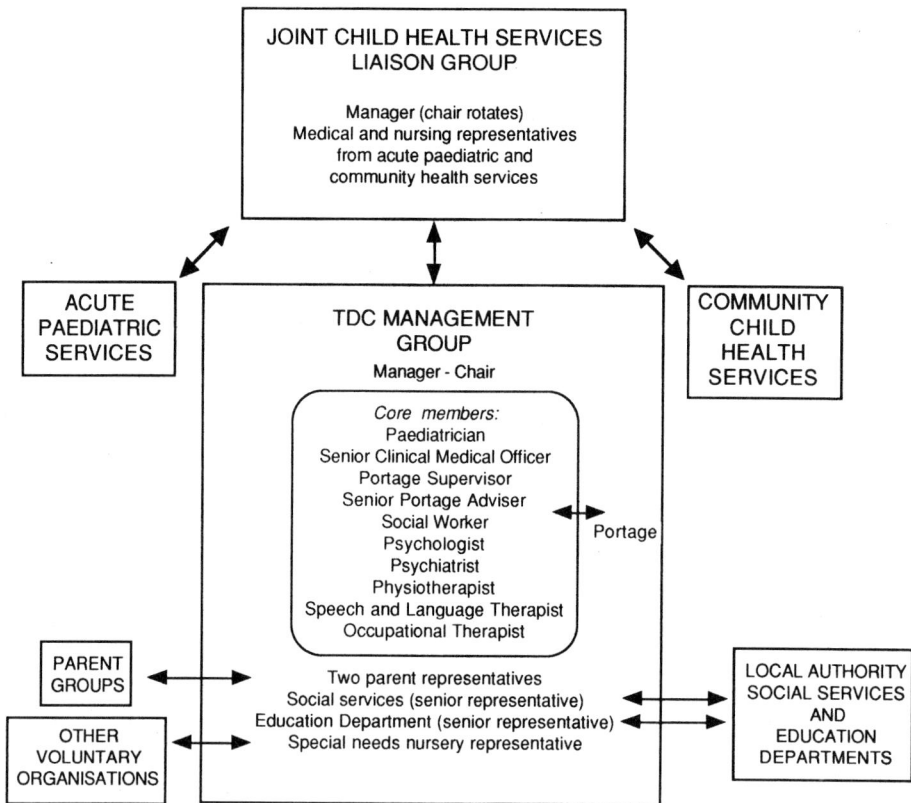

Fig. 4.1. Management structure of a Team for Disabled Children and their Families (TDC).

outside the team to the relevant professional organisation. Our own system of management and relationships is depicted in Figure 4.1.

Other teams function within larger groups of professionals, incorporating more therapists, teachers and others. The advantage of having a core group is that by keeping the numbers to a minimum the children and families are exposed to a limited number of people at any one consultation. Families are often intimidated by large numbers of apparent spectators, especially at their first introduction to the team. The core team system enhances trust and confidence between team members and gives a much closer identification of abilities and responsibilities. It is also more efficient economically for conferences with particular patients to involve fewer professionals. Teams incorporating larger groups of professionals may have the advantage of enabling more people to feel part of the team, but larger groups are more difficult to manage and responsibilities become more confused. Furthermore, most district health authorities are hard pushed to find adequate numbers of therapists to service the identified needs of the population, and involvement of large numbers of therapists in multidisciplinary assessments may be seen by management as an inappropriate use of professional time. Most teams therefore operate on a core or nucleus style. They perform comprehensive assessments gathering information over a period of time and when all the relevant information is available they formulate therapeutic intervention programmes. This process promotes the ability to keep a child disability register and update it at intervals. The most usual composition of the core team is shown in Table 4.1.The leader of the team is usually a senior clinical medical officer (SCMO) or consultant paediatrician (Table 4.2).

In time in the UK it is hoped that this role will be assumed by a consultant community paediatrician. The core of the team will usually include a social worker, nurse, physiotherapist, educational or clinical psychologist, and sometimes a speech therapist or occupational therapist. In Europe and the USA rehabilitationists (consultants in rehabilitation medicine) would lead the team or be represented. In the UK there is a significant need for more representation in teams from teachers and child psychiatrists.

One member of the team should be responsible for receiving referrals—usually the SCMO or paediatrician—who will decide whether the referral is appropriate for the team or should be dealt with at least initially in a general paediatric clinic. Often a preview, at a general paediatric clinic appointment, or in a special long first appointment with the paediatrician, will allow ground work to be done by establishing a relationship with the child and family and getting the basic history, family history and the parents' expectations clear before a multidisciplinary assessment. The paediatrician can then be sure that the essential members of the team will be present on the day that patient comes to the TDC appointment.

This style also allows the parents to identify with the team leader before being, as many might see it, 'challenged' by the whole group. Probably the next most important role within the team is that of the social worker: s/he will need to observe the transactions between the family and the other professionals; pick up spoken and unspoken fears, anxieties, doubts and uncertainties; and at an opportune moment, maybe after the consultation has finished, be available to explore those areas with the parents. Also, they will be a great help to the parents with claiming various allowances and benefits, and putting them in touch with the relevant statutory and voluntary organisations. If the team has compiled written information, such as a 'helping booklet' which outlines the services available locally, the social worker may be the best person to present this to the parents. In many cases the social worker will have become involved with the family before visiting the team. S/he may have been present at the initial diagnosis and breaking of bad news, or may have received a referral from the community social worker or other agency prior to the consultation. In the UK the medical social worker is now a member of the community social services department rather than a health authority employee.

If the core team has a psychologist, his or her professional skills can be used not only in formulating an educational plan, but also in looking at family interactions and relationships and, often more importantly, giving an objective view of the relationship between the team members and the family. The dynamics of relationships within the team will be another concern of the psychologist and social worker. They can support team members when they have doubts and anxieties concerning their own professional abilities and judgements.

41

TABLE 4.1
Make-up of the core team of District Handicap Teams (DHTs)*

	Number of units	% of units (N = 126)	% of DHTs (N = 94)
Social worker	94	74.6	100.0
Paediatrician	88	69.8	93.6
Senior clinical medical officer	74	58.7	78.7
Educational psychologist	68	54.0	72.3
Speech therapist	67	53.2	71.3
Physiotherapist	66	52.4	70.2
Health visitor	64	50.8	68.1
Nurse	51	40.5	54.3
Occupational therapist	42	33.3	44.7
Teacher	35	27.8	37.2
Clinical psychologist	30	23.8	31.9
Doctor	17	13.5	18.1
Psychologist	13	10.3	13.8
Senior medical officer	12	9.5	12.8
Nursery nurse	9	7.1	9.6
Psychiatrist	8	6.4	8.5
Audiologist	6	4.8	6.4
Clinical medical officer	6	4.8	6.4
Unit administrator	5	4.0	5.3
Consultant physician (mental handicap)	5	4.0	5.3
Orthoptist	5	4.0	5.3
Principal medical officer	4	3.2	4.3
Education welfare officer	3	2.4	3.2
Adviser in special education	3	2.4	3.2
Administrative assistant	3	2.4	3.2
Divisional social service officer	3	2.4	3.2
Specialist in community medicine	2	1.6	2.1
Director of nursing services	2	1.6	2.1
Representative from MENCAP†	2	1.6	2.1
Divisional nursing officer	2	1.6	2.1
Dietician	1	0.8	1.1
School medical officer	1	0.8	1.1
Specialist careers officer	1	0.8	1.1
Group therapist	1	0.8	1.1
Divisional medical officer	1	0.8	1.1
Dental officer	1	0.8	1.1
Assistant divisional education officer	1	0.8	1.1
Developmental officer	1	0.8	1.1
Psychiatric nurse	1	0.8	1.1

*Based on a questionnaire survey of child development centres in England and Wales. Of 126 units responding, 94 had some form of District Handicap Team, although interpretation of the findings was complicated by a lack of conformity in the use of terminology and in service structure (some centres, for instance, were not aware that the service they provided constituted that of a DHT).
†Royal Society for Mentally Handicapped Children and Adults.
Adapted from Bax and Whitmore (1985).

TABLE 4.2
Leadership of the team*

	Number of DHTs	% of DHTs (N = 94)*
Senior clinical medical officer	31	33.0
Consultant paediatrician	26	27.6
Paediatrician	4	4.2
Consultant community paediatrician	4	4.2
Senior medical officer	3	3.2
Consultant community physician	3	3.2
Specialist in community medicine	2	2.1
Associate specialist in paediatrics	2	2.1
Senior nurse	2	2.1
Senior social worker	2	2.1
Unit consultant	2	2.1
Medical coordinator	1	1.1
Liaison health visitor	1	1.1
Director of social services	1	1.1
Area education officer	1	1.1
Other	7	7.4

*See footnote, Table 4.1.
Adapted from Bax and Whitmore (1985).

Therapists working within the team have a role similar to that which they have outside the team: the assessment of needs and recommendations for therapy. However, within the team, therapists may often be consulted by other members rather than directly by the patient or parents and their role as teacher and adviser is an important one. Additionally, the therapists will learn skills from other members of the team which will enhance mutual confidence and respect without undermining professional standards or standing.

If early intervention programmes or specialised day care placements are available, one member of the team should have executive powers for admission to such facilities or at least act as the final common pathway for the referral. It is also important to know at any time how many places are available on such programmes so that the parents can be given up-to-date information, rather than being disappointed that a vacancy is not readily available after promises made by a team member remote from the programme. In a well established team different team members will assume various supporting roles not necessarily linked with their professional status and training.

It is important that the team for disabled children is not there just to organise assessment and therapies for disabled children, but that it also has a role in the prospective management of children and their families until such time as it is felt that the comprehensive umbrella of the service is no longer required.

Relationships with other organisations
Education
The team by nature will have relationships with other organisations. One of the most

important will be with the local education department. In most teams this function is fulfilled by the SCMO or by the consultant community paediatrician. S/he will be familiar with the local special education services and the necessary legislation for assessing children with special educational needs. In the UK the process of assessing whether a child has special educational needs—called 'statementing'—makes it important for this person to have a good working relationship with the relevant educational officer so that the resolution of difficult issues can be achieved without undue bureaucracy. Often the paediatrician, the consultant community paediatrician and the senior clinical medical officer will attend some of the special schools and thus develop relationships with the teaching staff and psychologists. If these relationships exist, the team will make realistic rather than idealistic demands on the education department and other services.

Psychiatry

If there is no psychiatrist as a core member of the team, links will need to be forged between the team and the local psychiatric service for children and families. This can be done in joint consultations as described by Sturge (1989), or by having a member of the child and family psychiatric service providing sessions in the child development centre.

Sturge describes the practices in child psychiatry and child psychiatric joint work, and liaison work with paediatrics. Concerning the latter, he underlines the need to establish at the point of referral, firstly the expectation of the referral, secondly the degree of collaboration needed, and thirdly, areas of responsibility. He details the functions of obtaining an opinion, consultation, joint work, parallel work and handovers, and how these different functions should be identified for different categories of problem. He also has observations on tertiary referrals in paediatrics, the difficulties in identifying continuing responsibility, and the misnomer of shared care between a paediatrician and the tertiary referral psychiatric service.

Liaison is promoted if all the services are under the same roof, again for cross fertilisation of ideas and recognition of the skills of the different disciplines. A very significant number of children attending TDCs have behavioural and conduct disorders, but only a minority of teams have psychiatrists as part of their core membership. Development of a psychiatric liaison service is outlined by Black *et al.* (1990).

Graham (1984) has pointed out that referrals to a psychiatric consultation service are less necessary when there is regular contact between specialists. Oke and Mayer (1991) conducted a survey of staff attitudes to referrals to child psychiatry and, in a questionnaire given to paediatricians and child psychiatrists, explored the type of problems and factors which might negatively influence referral. They noted that when there was a significant difference between child psychiatry staff and paediatricians it was always the child psychiatrists who were in favour of the referral and the paediatricians who were against it. One possible explanation for these findings was that paediatricians and child psychiatrists may have different ideas about the problems. It is likely that paediatricians would see a broad range in the severity of these cases, but the child psychiatric staff might see only the more severe cases. Another possible cause of those differences might have been the apparent lack of communication between the two departments. Concerning non-referral, both departments strongly agreed that inadequate communication was a reason for this. Oke and Mayer advocate more active attempts at communication between the two groups, with joint ward rounds or clinical meetings, more consultative work and more mutual education in meetings, saying that this would reduce the perceived need for many of the referrals. They also suggest a jointly formulated referral policy.

Social services
The team will not only have a relationship with the social services through the medical social worker: the social services agency may also require information concerning particular children in order to provide aids for home living and structural modifications to the home, and these enquiries are usually addressed to the consultant in charge. Additionally, the team may recommend children to facilities run by the local social services department, such as day care nurseries or residential nurseries, and it is important that close relationships are maintained. Occasionally case conferences will need to be convened between team members and social services departments when there is suspicion of neglect or abuse within the family, especially since it is becoming clearer that disabled children are more vulnerable to abuse than their ordinary peers (Russell 1992): indeed, abuse may be the cause of disability (Lask *et al.* 1991).

Community learning disability team (or equivalent)
Most TDCs maintain strong links with their local community learning disability team (CLDT) and such teams usually take over the management of children with learning difficulties when they leave school. CLDTs may have particular areas of strength, such as a good psychology service, which can be used for children with severe behavioural problems. The Court Report (1976) recommended that CLDTs should confine their activities to their adult clientele. Bax and Whitmore (1991) found that 65 per cent of CLDTs saw children. It is important that the DHT or TDC should keep the CLDT informed of children who are likely to graduate into the adult services and do this well in advance of the transfer of care. The CLDT will often require access to the DHT or TDC register in order to plan services effectively. The social services departments will also need access to the register since in the UK and many other countries there are statutory responsibilities to inform social services departments and education departments of children with special needs.

Voluntary organisations
Recently there has been a large increase in the number of voluntary organisations concerned with specific syndrome groups. Some organisations in the UK, such as the Research Trust for Metabolic Disease in Children, include a large group of mainly very rare disorders. Others are more global, *e.g.* MENCAP (the Royal Society for Mentally Handicapped Children and Adults), which caters for all people with learning difficulties. Still others are very specific, *e.g.* LINK ('Let's Increase Neurofibromatosis Knowledge'). In the UK, the Contact a Family (CaF) Directory (1991) is a comprehensive source for these groups.

Some families may wish to become involved with two or three organisations which have a bearing on their child's problem. Others will receive information concerning the organisation and make no effort to become involved. Often parents are helped by receiving information from these sources, but only a limited number become active participants in the group. For very rare disorders the numbers of involved families will be small, making meetings difficult because of the distance between affected families. Often, once put in touch with a family with similar problems, there will be correspondence and telephone calls to maintain contact (see Chapter 9). There are clear advantages in parents finding out from these groups more about their child's condition. However, there are times when they need the local services and should realise that the two functions can be complementary and not mutually exclusive. Specialised groups involved with rare conditions should not try to take over the general services locally by making inappropriate demands. They need to recognise that the majority of special needs children require a rather general type of service.

Those of us who have informed parents about these groups over the years know that not all families wish to be associated with support groups, some because they are not naturally 'club oriented' and some because they are not comfortable with a particular group for whatever reason. Many will find the local services adequate and just keep their knowledge of progress topped up by a tenuous relationship with these organisations. The local branches of national specialised voluntary organisations tend to wax and wane, not just in proportion to the number of children with the relevant disorder, but more in relationship to the energies and motivations of the parents involved and the ages of their children. Parents with younger children and greater expectations appear to have most energy.

The TDC has a responsibility to be aware of these groups, and there is now in the UK a statutory responsibility to inform parents of the appropriate voluntary organisation(s) as soon as the child's needs are known. Various members of the TDC, for instance the medical social worker, may be involved in setting up parent support groups, though they do not necessarily have a continued involvement once these are functioning. Additionally, voluntary organisations and support groups may have information and recommendations to make to TDCs to help them improve their services and sensitivity in handling patients and their families.

Team dynamics

In his 'Tower of Babel' address to the 30th Annual Meeting of the American Academy for Cerebral Palsy and Developmental Medicine, Pearson (1983) referred to the different languages of various professionals and their differing levels of training: different disciplines have knowledge bases expanding at different rates; different professional organisations change the rules; coping with changes in legislation is a major problem; and professionals have different perceptions of their own roles and those of others. He offered a 'matrix' for interdisciplinary collaboration (Table 4.3).

Pearson commented, 'Being comfortable in one's own professional rôle allows one to be more flexible in accepting and integrating the views of others, obviating the tendency to practice one-upmanship. 'Professional hierarchies' can become barriers to effective collaboration, since some doctoral-level professionals seem to have trouble accepting the fact that they can gain important information from, for example, a bachelor-level physical therapist or educator'. He voiced a concern regarding professional territoriality and

TABLE 4.3
A 'matrix' for interdisciplinary collaboration: the 'process'

Professionalism	Communication	Philosophical and psychological factors
Attitudes and values systems	Language barriers: jargon, acronyms	Leadership styles
Technical skills		Case management
Theoretical framework	Common body of knowledge	Team management
Territoriality	Monitoring system and behavioural objectives	Emotional climate: trust–respect–openness
Pre-defined roles	'Process' meetings	Decision-making shared responsibility
Professional hierarchies	Formal/informal channels of communication	
		Management priorities

Adapted from Pearson (1983).

suggested a core curriculum for all professionals involved in order to achieve a common body of knowledge and language, thus promoting a better level of understanding of the requirements of other members of the team. Pearson made suggestions for validating the diagnostic statements of the team and recommendations for formal and informal channels for communication between members. He also covered team management, suggesting that the leadership of the team should be decided on the basis of the specific team-task. This is an interesting idea, but not realistic in most cases.

Price (1989), a physiotherapist who has studied team work within ambulant specialist care, made 210 enquiries of 35 units in Sweden. She found that lack of time was the most common obstacle to a meaningful meeting, rather than professional language, poor punctuality, poor meeting discipline or too large a group.

A hearing for team members' points of view was gained in 86 per cent of cases; 54 per cent felt that they could freely question the views of other members and only 6 per cent did so seldom or never; while 65 per cent of respondents failed to answer the question 'do you feel that some professional colleagues have a tendency to dominate team work?' Physiotherapists and doctors were thought to be the most dominating.

Bailey (1984) proposed a three-dimensional model of conceptualising problems in the functioning of the interdisciplinary team (Fig. 4.2). He points out that team growth is a developmental process. Teams are made up of individuals, and sometimes dysfunctioning may result from interpersonal problems or subsystems within the team. The team may be conceptualised as a functioning unit, and some problems are the result of whole team dysfunction. He pictured the perspectives of team development as four levels, from unidisciplinary (you alone, your clinic), through multidisciplinary, with each discipline remaining independent, to interdisciplinary, where outcome is advanced through interactive effort, and finally to transdisciplinary. The latter, according to Lyon and Lyon (1980), has three characteristics. The first is the joint team approach in which it is assumed

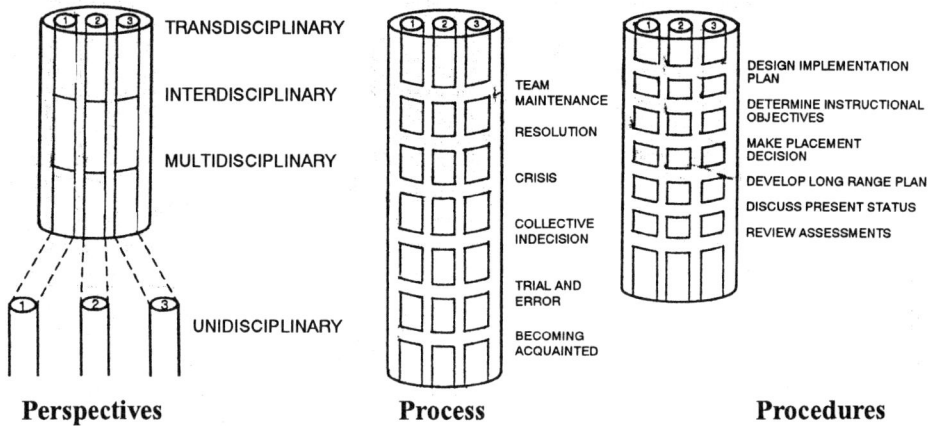

Perspectives   **Process**   **Procedures**

Fig. 4.2. Examples of models of team development. (Adapted by permission from Bailey 1984.)

that the team must perform the various services together. In the second, a staff development approach is taken in which the expertise of individual team members is recognised and used to train other team members. The third characteristic is role release, in which the roles and responsibilities are shared by more than one team member.

After describing the evolution of the transdisciplinary team, Bailey went on to describe the process in a developmental sequence of six stages as suggested by Lowe and Herranen (1982):

In Stage I, Becoming Acquainted, team members first come together as a team. This stage frequently is characterized by hierarchical group structures, autocratic leadership, polite and impersonal inter-actions, and low overall team productivity. In Stage II, Trial and Error, the team begins to try to work together toward a common goal. Team members align themselves with one or two other team members, and factions may occur. Role conflict and ambiguity become problems as team members attempt to co-ordinate efforts. In Stage III, Collective Indecision,

the group attempts to avoid direct conflict and achieve equilibrium . . . decisions are made by default and are characterised by the assumption that responsibilities are shared when, in fact, they are not. There is no group norm for accountability and thus little is accomplished. [Lowe and Herranen 1982.]

In Stage IV, Crisis, some event forces the team's hand. Team members express considerable emotion, and they begin to realize the importance of their mission, although overall team productivity may be low. In Stage V, Resolution, the group makes a concerted effort to work together as a team. "It is characterized by open communication, shared leadership, decision-making and responsibility" [Lowe and Herranen, 1982]. In Stage VI, Team Maintenance, "the paramount driving force finally becomes the client's . . . needs" [Lowe and Herranen, 1982].

This sequence compares well with that described by Handy (1985) where becoming acquainted is likened to *forming*; trial and error, to *storming*; collective indecision, crisis and resolution to *norming*; and team maintenance to *performing*.

Forming

The group is not yet a team but a set of individuals. This stage is characterised by talk about the purpose of the group, the definition and the title of the group, and its composition, leadership pattern and life-span. At this stage, too, each individual tends to want to establish his or her personal identity within the group and make some individual impression.

Storming

Most groups go through a conflict stage when the preliminary, and often false, consensus on purposes, on leadership and other roles, and on norms of work and behaviour is challenged and re-established. At this stage a lot of personal agendas are revealed and a certain amount of interpersonal hostility is generated. If successfully handled, this period of storming leads to a new and more realistic setting of objectives, procedures and norms. This stage is particularly important for testing the norms of trust in the group.

Norming

The group needs to establish norms and practices concerning when and how it should work; how it should take decisions; and what type of behaviour, what level of work, and what degree of openness, trust and confidence is appropriate. At this stage there will be a lot of tentative experimentation by individuals to test the temperature of the group and to measure the appropriate level of commitment.

Performing

Only when the three previous stages have been successfully completed will the group be at full maturity and be able to be fully and sensibly productive. Some kind of performance will be achieved at all stages of development but it is likely to be impeded by the other processes of growth and by individual agendas. In many periodic committees the issues of leadership, or of the objectives and purpose of the group, are recurring topics that crop up in every meeting in some form or other, seriously hindering the true work of the group.

A further stage, not proposed by Handy, could be *reforming*, where the team is able to take on new members and change direction according to circumstances.

Handy was considering groups working in commerce and industry, but the principles apply to any group with a common task when the nature of the task, criteria for effectiveness, salience of the task and clarity of the task are understood. As teams evolve it may be difficult to identify these stages because over a long period of time they may be happening insidiously (and for well established, efficiently functioning teams they probably have no relevance), but they are important stages to consider when evolving new teams for specialist functions.

Further, Bailey (1984) went on to describe team subsystems, taking an ideal model based on the assumption that the ideal team is one in which: (i) the leader is present but acts as a member of the team; (ii) each team member is relatively equal in power and influence; and (iii) conflict and disagreements are based on substantive issues rather than personality conflicts. Examples of team subsystem dysfunction are illustrated in Figure 4.3.

Similarly, Bailey dealt with whole team functioning on a graphic basis (Fig. 4.4), and

IDEAL TEAM

UNDERPERFORMING TEAM

AMBIGUOUS ROLES

OVERSTRUCTURED TEAM

DISORGANIZED TEAM

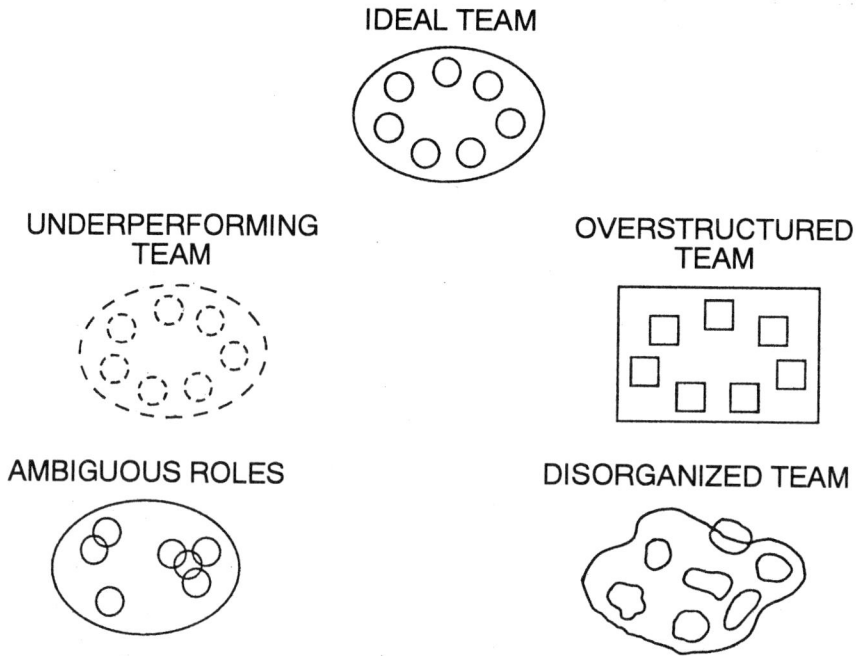

Fig. 4.3. Team subsystem function and dysfunction. (Adapted by permission from Bailey 1984.)

it has to be recognised and remembered that each team is composed of unique individuals in a unique setting.

Handy (1985) has written about leadership and leadership theories and on the workings of groups. One useful concept of leadership, not often quoted, is the 'Helicopter factor' where the ability of the leader 'to rise above the particulars of a situation and perceive it in its relations to the overall environment' is a key attribute.

On leadership and doctors, Smith (1992) quotes Professor Warren Bennis:

"Leading doctors is a bit like herding cats . . . Doctors are independent and autonomous, and the very reason they selected medicine was because of their fierce desire for autonomy. The idea of a physician-manager is an oxymoron," said Professor Bennis. "But some of the best administrators I've ever met have come out of medicine. I would let them run anything. They get from medicine a sense of system. They don't go for false simplifications. They know how to intervene without causing harm. All of the best principles of medicine should work in management.

"But most doctors have a hard time with management. I've taught a lot of physicians, and nothing in their education has prepared them for the technology of cooperation. They are self absorbed and used to personal intervention rather than working in teams. They don't have that literacy of teamwork, collaboration, and empowering other people."

"What is the job of a leader?" I asked Professor Bennis.

"Simply put, it is to show direction and generate trust. When you ask people what they want from leaders they use words like vision, dream, direction, mission, goal, and purpose, but also credibility."

50

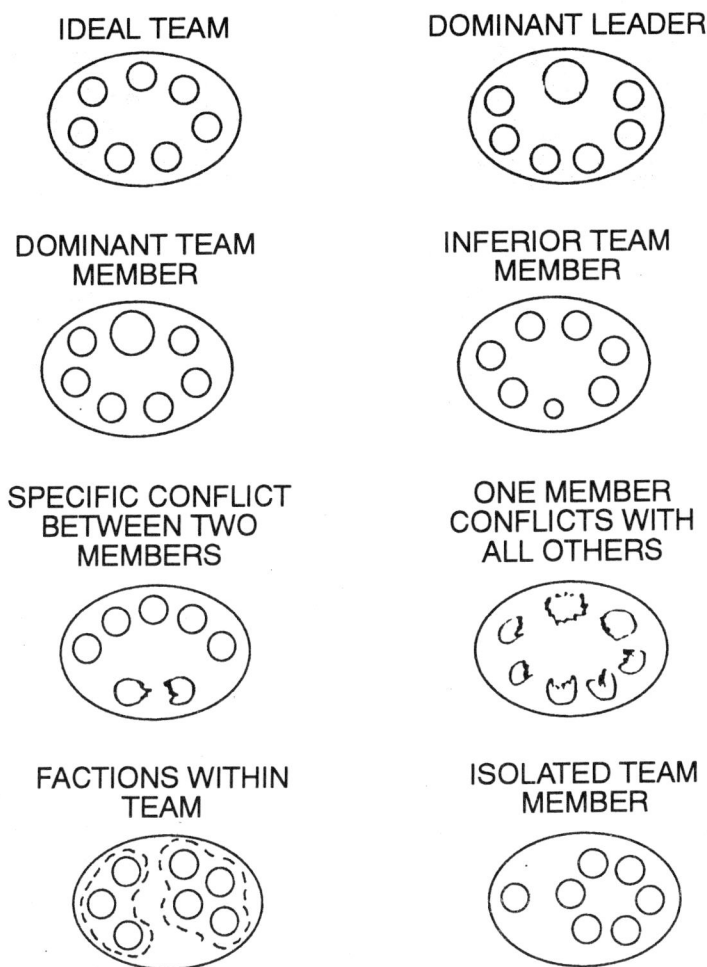

IDEAL TEAM

DOMINANT LEADER

DOMINANT TEAM MEMBER

INFERIOR TEAM MEMBER

SPECIFIC CONFLICT BETWEEN TWO MEMBERS

ONE MEMBER CONFLICTS WITH ALL OTHERS

FACTIONS WITHIN TEAM

ISOLATED TEAM MEMBER

Fig. 4.4. Whole team function and dysfunction. (Adapted by permission from Bailey 1984.)

Further help is available from Gale and Grant (1990). They have generated guidelines for those who wish to affect change in a medical context. These are derived from wide-based consultations with doctors mainly in education and management spheres and constructed using their own deep experience of the change process. Their summary of the process for medical change is shown in Table 4.4. As can be seen, each of the ten core activities needs to be considered carefully, and at each stage consultation and feedback is required.

Team leadership is an issue which can be endlessly debated. Ultimately communications within and without the team are required, and it is usually one individual who is

TABLE 4.4
A model of medical change

Professional characteristics and styles	Core activities	Tactical choices and styles
Consultation	1 ESTABLISH THE NEED	Lobbying, consultation, conjunction of circumstances
Demonstration	2 POWER TO ACT	Key people, ownership, harnessing committees, authority/borrowed power, political/external power, personal position, local environment
Evolution Ownership	3 DESIGN THE INNOVATION	Feasible?, resources, timing, timescale, involvement, directive/elective, scale, degree, predicting pathways and barriers, winners and losers
Power to hinder	4 CONSULT	Appropriateness, leadership, teamwork, talking and explaining
Commitment	5 PUBLICISE THE CHANGE WIDELY	Presentation, vision, amending proposals, communication
Energy/enthusiasm	6 AGREE DETAILED PLANS	Detailed plans
Motives	7 IMPLEMENT	Demonstration projects, scheming/bypassing, implementation strategy, opportunism, pathways and barriers to change
	8 PROVIDE SUPPORT	Resistance, overcoming difficulties, objections, maintaining change
	9 MODIFY PLANS	Compensation, modifications
	10 EVALUATE OUTCOMES	Evaluation strategy

Gale and Grant (1990).

responsible for generating summarising reports and acting in the capacity of link-person with other relevant organisations. Some teams prefer this role to be a rotating responsibility, but usually one person will take it on or be able to delegate it to another. This will very much depend upon local circumstances, but the team which has insights into the processes described above will be best able to influence its own function.

REFERENCES

Bailey, D.B. (1984) 'A triaxial model of the interdisciplinary team and group process.' *Exceptional Children*, **51**, 17–25.

Bax, M.C.O., Whitmore, K. (1985) *District Handicap Teams: Structure, Function and Relationships. Report to DHSS*. London: Community Paediatric Research Unit, Westminster Children's Hospital.

—— —— (1991) 'District handicap teams in England: 1983-8.' *Archives of Disease in Childhood*, **66**, 656–664.

Black, D., McFadyen, A., Broster, G. (1990) 'Development of a psychiatric liaison service.' *Archives of Disease in Childhood*, **65**, 1373–1375.

Contact a Family (1991) *CaF Directory of Specific Conditions and Rare Syndromes in Children with their Family Support Networks*. London: CaF.

Court Report (1976) *Fit for the Future. Report of the Committee on Child Health Services. Vol. 1. Cmnd. 6684*. London: HMSO.

Gale, R., Grant, J. (1990) *Guidelines for Change in Postgraduate and Continuing Medical Education*. London: Joint Centre for Educational Research and Development in Medicine.

Graham, P. (1984) 'Paediatric referral to a child psychiatrist.' *Archives of Disease in Childhood*, **59**, 1103–1105.

Handy, C.B. (1985) *Understanding Organisations*. London: Penguin.

Lask, B., Britten, C., Kroll, L., Magagna, J., Tranter, M. (1991) 'Children with pervasive refusal.' *Archives of Disease in Childhood*, **66**, 866–869.

Lowe, J.I., Herranen, M. (1982) 'Understanding teamwork: another look at the concepts.' *Social Work in Health Care*, **7**(2), 1–11.

Lyon, S., Lyon, G. (1980) 'Team functioning and staff development: a rôle release approach to providing integrated educational services for severely handicapped students.' *Journal of the Association for the Severely Handicapped*, **5**, 250–263.

Oke, S., Mayer, R. (1991) 'Referrals to child psychiatry—a survey of staff attitudes.' *Archives of Disease in Childhood*, **66**, 862–865.

Pearson, P.H. (1983) 'The interdisciplinary team process, or the professionals' Tower of Babel.' *Developmental Medicine and Child Neurology*, **25**, 390–395.

Price, E. (1989) 'Paediatric habilitation—a study on teamwork within ambulant specialist care.' *Paper presented to the 1st Meeting of the European Academy of Childhood Disability, Oxford*.

Rosenbloom, L. (1985) 'District handicap teams. Service models.' *Paper presented to The Spastics Society Medical Education and Information Unit*.

Russell, P. (1992) 'Caring for children living away from home.' *In:* McCarthy, G.T. (Ed.) *Physical Disability in Childhood. An Interdisciplinary Approach to Management*. Edinburgh: Churchill Livingstone, pp. 507–524

Smith, R. (1992) 'Leadership and doctors.' *British Medical Journal*, **305**, 137–138.

Sturge J.C. (1989) 'Joint work in paediatrics: a child psychiatry perspective.' *Archives of Disease in Childhood*, **64**, 155–158.

5
IS A CHILD DEVELOPMENT CENTRE (CDC) NECESSARY?

The argument for having a 'bricks and mortar' building as a centre for the TDC is much stronger when service provision is being threatened by financial constraints than at more favourable times. If a building exists and is being fully used properly for service provision, it is much more difficult for managers to dispose of it or use it for something else than it is for them to postpone or cancel the reappointment of personnel who leave. That is not to say that the two things are mutually exclusive because they are not. However, if a service is run on a peripatetic basis the loss of two or three staff members will not be as apparent as it would if they worked within and from a centre. In other words a service run from a secure base is a more secure service.

Bax and Whitmore (1991a) recommended that every district should have a CDC and they highlighted its essential features by updating the Court Report's (1976) original recomendations as follows:

(1) The child development centre should be closely associated with the district general hospital but equally committed to providing a peripatetic service in satellite premises (especially in rural areas and in selected schools).

(2) Given this assurance, local education and social service authorities should be prepared to enter into joint arrangements for funding and staffing the child development centre.

(3) The child development centre should initially be able to cater for the needs of all children [under 16 years—see Bax and Whitmore 1991b], and for older children in the absence of adequate, similar facilities for disabled adolescents.

(4) The child development centre should be able to provide initial assessment and treatment for children with any kind of disorder, leaving community mental handicap teams to concentrate on the continuing special needs of mentally handicapped adolescents and adults.

(5) To meet this demand, the child development centre should have regular weekly sessions from a consultant community paediatrician, a liaison health visitor, another nurse, a social worker familiar with the needs of disabled children, a psychologist with expertise in the cognitive assessment of disabled children and the management of emotional and behavioural difficulties, a teacher, a physiotherapist, speech therapist, and an occupational therapist, all of whom should be experienced in working with such children.

(6) The child development centre should also have at least one session a week from a child psychiatrist and regular (though not necessarily weekly) sessions from children's orthopaedic, ophthalmic, and audiology specialists.

(7) The referral of children to a child development centre should normally be initiated by a general practitioner, a paediatrician, or another medical specialist, but the centre should also adopt the policy of open referral from parents and any professional attending the child.

(8) As well as providing a clinical service, a child development centre should be prepared and equipped to act as a district resource and information centre for disabled children, and to contribute

to the inservice training of all professionals in the district who may play a part in the care of disabled children.

(9) The child development centre should take part in the district's epidemiological studies relating to disabled children and help to monitor the service it provides.

Bax and Whitmore (1985) found that 192 districts all put different interpretations on the constitution or placement of District Handicap Teams as proposed by Court (1976). These ranged from 82 where a DHT was functioning in a CDC, to 25 with no DHT or CDC. 50 per cent of the DHTs practice on hospital premises where there were often problems with parking and staffing. Between 1973 and 1983 the number of health authorities with special centres for disabled children had more than doubled, but barely half of them seemed to be functioning as a full DHT.

There is an argument that if the CDC exists, then assessments will tend to be done there rather than at home, but some workers feel that the domiciliary developmental assessment is more valid than the one performed at the centre. This issue has recently been explored by Rosenbaum et al. (1990) who state that despite the obvious logic of offering service to people in their own homes, many aspects of the assessment and treatment of young children with developmental disabilities have not been evaluated critically to assess their efficacy and cost effectiveness. A pilot study indicated that both parents and therapists expressed strong preference for the therapist's first assessment of developmentally disabled children to be conducted at home. They caution, however, that some families might find a home assessment threatening or intrusive and prefer to go to the professionals. There are also costs in time and money incurred by professionals visiting children at home, and administrative proscriptions on expenditure could inhibit a new approach to service.

Rosenbaum et al. proposed three specific hypotheses:

(1) Children will be more comfortable in their homes than in an unfamiliar clinic, and therefore will perform in a manner more typical of their daily function.
(2) In the home, therapists will be able to assess a wider range of a child's functions (communication, activities of daily living, motor, play) and the home environment than would be possible at the clinic.
(3) Parents will feel more relaxed in their own home, and more satisfied with an assessment performed there, than will parents attending an unfamiliar clinic.

The results of this study show, with regard to hypothesis one, that 'There were no statistically significant differences in the rates of 'typical' behaviour between home and clinic groups as judged by parents.'

For hypothesis two, 'Therapists felt that they had obtained adequate information about all areas of their assessment, both at home or at the clinic, except for the knowledge of the child's environment. . . Children's communication was more often assessed directly at home . . . than at the clinic . . . although adequate information had been obtained by a combination of observation and parental report in both settings. . . There were virtually no differences between groups regarding activities of daily living, motor function or play.'

For hypothesis three, 'Parents of children seen at home expressed much greater preference for home assessment . . . than did the parents seen at the clinic. . . There were no other differences between parents in the two groups regarding any aspects of the process or content of the assessment.'

This study is concerned with therapist assessment and could probably be extrapolated to clinical medical officers or their equivalents in other communities. Also there will be differences in the rural/urban mix of communities which will influence the relative home/CDC benefit relationships.

Other activities outside the CDC include visits by professionals to children in their nurseries, special schools or residential homes. The professional is acting in these sessions on behalf of the TDC and there needs to be communication with other relevant members. Sometimes school-age children and their parents will prefer to be seen at school. Others will prefer to visit the centre and this often puts an extra load on the service during school holidays because that is when these children's parents prefer them to be seen.

Generally the TDC does meet in a CDC but some of its activities, such as in education, could be in the Postgraduate Medical Centre or, for planning, in the offices of management. If proper facilities exist in a CDC then managers will be attracted to it and money may follow. It will also attract the other statutory and voluntary bodies in addition to patients and parents. If the TDC is operating on a core basis it is convenient for the building to have accommodation for other individuals involved in evaluation and therapy so that they can be on hand in the same building thus promoting informal as well as formal exchanges. It is also essential to have secretarial and clerical support in the centre. Notes must be available and registers accessible along with relevant administrative and appointment systems.

A base, therefore, with a central office and consulting and conferencing facilities, and appropriate equipment for therapy is the minimum requirement. It is an advantage to have adequate waiting areas and play rooms adjacent. The centre should be welcoming and available for parent–user groups. It should not necessarily be based on the medical or clinic model; other facilities including a library, a teaching area, a kitchen, a soft play area, a special needs information (or resource) centre and a quiet room or hiding place would complete most people's requirements.

Some centres will have the good fortune to be able to house a special needs nursery on the site. This is much more likely if the centre is based on education department premises than in a health establishment. If the nursery is within the CDC, therapists and others have ample opportunity to observe the children, and to have day to day contact and exchanges with nursery staff. In this way, those making assessments of the children obtain a much more complete profile of their abilities and problems than is obtainable from a single assessment and written reports from care staff.

It is, of course, very helpful to the families of disabled children if most of their requirements can be met under one roof, in a centre with which they can identify. However, this does risk encouraging overdependence in some cases, and suitable safeguards need to be taken if this is anticipated. It also gives the professionals a base and a meeting point where they can exchange views and experiences in informal corridor or coffee room style, as well as in the more formal structured consultations.

A CDC is usually the place where regional specialists such as visiting neurologists or geneticists will conduct their joint clinics with local professionals and it will allow them to meet the rest of the team formally and informally from time to time (see Appendix 1, p. 104).

The success of a CDC depends upon its ability to motivate parents, to be a source of information and help, and to provide a warm and hopeful environment. It requires a management committee with a written statement of policy, aims and objectives. This body will have parent representatives and be able to produce annual reports of activity and future plans. (For an outline of our own management system, see Fig. 4.1, p. 40.)

REFERENCES

Bax, M.C.O., Whitmore, K. (1985) *District Handicap Teams: Structure, Function and Relationships. Report to DHSS.* London: Community Paediatric Research Unit, Westminster Children's Hospital.
—— —— (1991a) 'District Handicap Teams in England: 1983–8.' *Archives of Disease in Childhood,* **66**, 656–664.
—— ——(1991b) 'District Handicap Teams in England, 1983–8.' *Archives of Disease in Childhood,* **66**, 1103. *(Letter.)*
Court Report (1976) *Fit for the Future. Report of the Committee on Child Health Services. Vol. 1. Cmnd. 6684.* London: HMSO.
Rosenbaum, P., King, S., Toal, C., Puttaswamaiah, S., Durrell, K. (1990) 'Home or children's treatment centre: where should initial therapy assessments of children with disabilities be done?' *Developmental Medicine and Child Neurology,* **32**, 888–894.

6
THE CONSULTATION PROCESS

Referral or intake

Bax and Whitmore (1985) list the sources of referral to DHTs: of the units interviewed, 67 per cent named community health doctors; 63 per cent mentioned consultant paediatricians; 41 per cent mentioned general practitioners (GPs); 40 per cent mentioned neonatal follow-up, including special care baby units; and 37 per cent mentioned health visitors. It may well be that many GP referrals were initiated either by health visitors or by community doctors (my own experience is that GPs do not necessarily state that fact in their referring letters).

Bax and Whitmore commented that GPs did not make much contact with DHTs. However, the introduction in the UK of threshold payments to GPs for child health surveillance should mean that appropriate referrals will increase.

The term 'primary care team' is used in the UK to indicate the front line of health care. The front line includes the GP, the health visitor and other professionals. The health visitor in the UK is a registered nurse with additional training to equip her or him to provide an advice and support service for all parents and children. All GPs have a health visitor working with them. Community paediatricians are the secondary referral level, alongside the hospital paediatricians. Figure 6.1 shows how our referral system works.

In the USA and in other developed countries, children may be under the care of a paediatrician from birth. Indeed, the obstetrician may refer newborn babies to paediatricians whether there are problems or not. This means the paediatrician is responsible for the primary health care of all children—both normal and those with special needs—including immunisation, and general health and developmental examinations. To some extent this system applies also in continental Europe.

In developing countries there may be no primary care doctor or paediatrician, and it is usually health care workers of different levels of expertise and training who will identify children with special needs—usually at the parents' instigation—and refer them on to any intervention programme which may exist. Thorburn and Marfo (1990) describe the approaches to childhood disability in a broad spectrum of different socioeconomic backgrounds in developing countries.

A report from the Utrecht Research Centre on Child Health Care (de Winter *et al.* 1989) explored schemes for early detection of developmental disorders in young children. It revealed extreme variation in the frequency of developmental examinations amongst the 24 countries (20 of which were European) studied. Additionally, they detected significant gaps in the service. These were:

- lack of standardized system of E[arly] D[iagnosis] of developmental disorders
- lack of E.D. and screening methods/tools/equipment
- inadequate training of professionals (doctors and health workers)

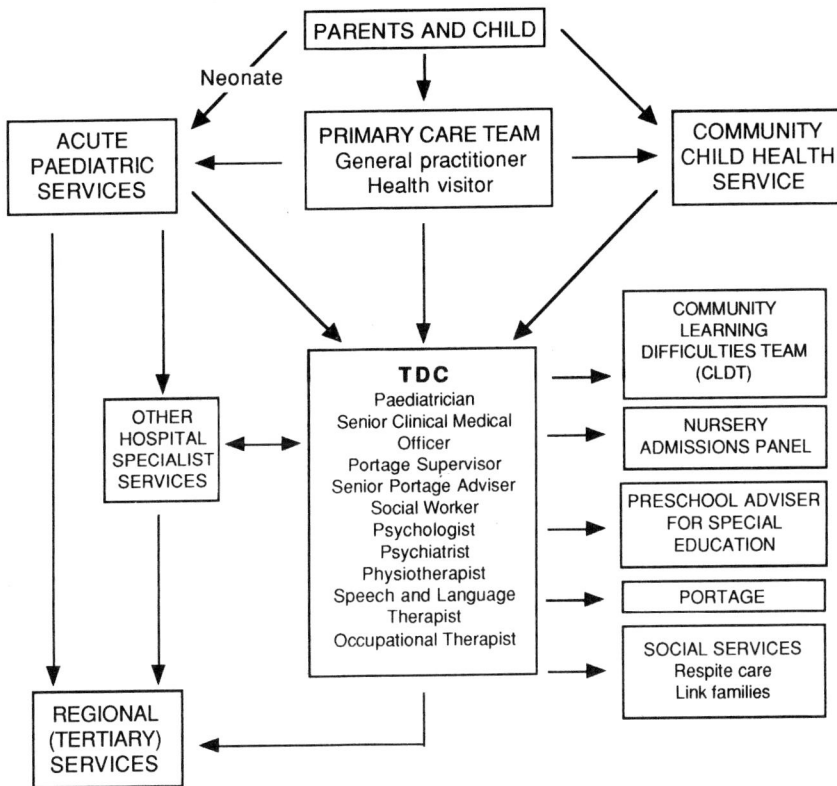

Fig. 6.1. Referral systems for a Team for Disabled Children and their Families (TDC).

- unenlightened attitude on behalf of professionals towards children with disorders
- inadequate cooperation between various disciplines of health visitors
- lack of/inadequate follow-up
- lack of professionals/resources/facilities, especially in rural areas
- inadequate/lack of research
- inadequate knowledge of parents with respect to normal/abnormal development and existing facilities; lack of support for parents
- lack of organized referral system
- lack of organized registration system
- time-lags between diagnosis (which often comes too late) and treatment
- lack of systematic screening for all children
- small screening-spectrum.

These findings are hardly surprising when consensus on the best methods for early detection of disability cannot be reached within even one country.

Hall *et al.* (1991) discuss the merits of early detection of disability. They point out that improved outcome is established when early detection is achieved in disorders such as phenylketonuria, hypothyroidism and congenital dislocation of the hip. They conclude that the evidence is equivocal for sensory neural hearing loss. Sometimes early diagnosis leads to genetic counselling which may prevent the birth of a child with the same disorder, *e.g.* muscular dystrophy.

Even if early diagnosis does not reduce the severity of the disability, appropriate intervention is thought to enable the child and family to cope with the disability more effectively by reducing parental frustration and isolation, and by helping the child make the most effective use of any functions and abilities that are preserved. Hall *et al.* highlight the fact that the most compelling reason for early diagnosis is that parents want it. Cunningham *et al.* (1984), Quine and Pahl (1987) and McConachie *et al.* (1988) have all provided evidence to support this contention, and personal experience confirms it. An early diagnosis must be accompanied by adequate counselling to facilitate adaptation and adjustment to the problems created by the disability and its disclosure.

Hall *et al.* suggest that the routine developmental examination of all children should be discontinued but assume that the existing surveillance of all children in the UK will proceed (see Chapter 2). The reasons given for this are that:

A large proportion of defects and disorders are detected in one of four ways:
(1)   the neonatal and six-week examinations;
(2)   follow-up of infants and children who have suffered various forms of trauma or illness affecting the nervous system;
(3)   detection by parents or relatives;
(4)   detection by playgroup leaders, nursery nurses, health visitors, and general practitioners in the course of their regular work.

Hall *et al.* further analyse the benefits of various 'screening' tests for impairments and disabilities and make recommendations for individual elements of 'screening' based on published results. These recommendations are, however, disputed by Bax and Whitmore (1990) who point out that Hall and colleagues take little account of the heterogeneity of urban populations and base their concepts on unsupported contentions about the ability of the majority of parents rather than the ability of all parents to bring their child's problems to professional attention.

It clearly should be part of the responsibility of a TDC to attempt to monitor whether it is receiving the appropriate number of referrals. Clinical audit can be employed to investigate, for instance, those children who, on reaching school entry, are found to have previously undiagnosed special needs or those children whose sensory neural hearing deficit is not diagnosed until two years of age or other indices of inefficient surveillance. This is an issue which should be dealt with at TDC management level: they should recommend appropriate changes and procedures to remedy the fault and monitor the expected improvement.

The referral letter to the TDC should be reviewed by a clinician before appointments are made. It is my practice to see babies or children with minor disability in a general paediatric clinic in the first instance. I see children with complex or profound problems at a special consultation lasting between half an hour and an hour so that all background information can be noted, and reports requested from other bodies, before the family comes to its first TDC appointment. This has a number of advantages over a direct referral to the team.

Firstly it allows a one-to-one relationship to develop between the paediatrician and the parents; secondly only one person is required to tabulate the history and obtain records from agencies previously involved; thirdly a paediatrician can best judge whether outstanding assessments need to be performed before the child attends the TDC. The first physical examination can be performed at this initial consultation in relative privacy. The parents' understanding of the problems at this point can also be explored. In this way comprehensive and up-to-date information about the child will be available at the first meeting with the team.

Having conducted this first consultation, the paediatrician will know whether the child really needs a TDC appointment and can often pre-empt this relatively labour intensive and expensive exercise if the problem is reasonably well defined and can be treated in a routine general paediatric clinic. On the other hand, if the paediatrician decides that the TDC is required, s/he can then be sure to obtain outstanding documentation of further or previous assessments before the first team consultation, and an appointment can be arranged timed to coincide with the availability of those things. Another possibility in some cases would be a referral to an independent agency, if special expertise is required.

Preparation

Our practice is to review the notes of children a week or two before the TDC consultation, whether they be new or follow-up patients. In this way the whole team can be briefed about the child; key members will already have received summarising letters following the original consultation; views of the members can be sought prior to the appointment; and the agenda for the consultation can, to a large extent, be predicted. This will include considering whether long time follow-up is likely to be necessary or whether it is probably a single consultation, and which team members need to be present. This avoids 'redundant players' at the consultation, which is important since parents may reasonably take exception to individuals with ill-defined or unstated roles being present.

Some teams send written information to parents of preschool children with developmental delay prior to their attendance at the CDC. Reed *et al.* (1993) have assessed the content of such material and make the following recommendations:

1   Written text should be assessed using the Flesch formulae (Flesch 1948, 1949) in order to ensure that it achieves a Human Interest Score of 'interesting' or 'very interesting', together with a Readability Score which predicts that it will be accessible to 75% of the population.

2   Staff should consider the inclusion of written text enquiring about the need for booklet translation in additional languages which represent the ethnicity of the population served by the CDC.

3   Staff should consider including photographs of children actively engaged in play and therapeutic activities. It seems important to show children from different ethnic backgrounds and to include both men and women involved in activities with children.

4   There should be consultation with parent consumers in order to elicit their views on the usefulness and acceptability of the text and format.

5   The results of this study suggest that the consumers would like more lengthy descriptions to inform them about what to expect from different members of staff.

The consultation

Often the first question to ask parents will be, 'Who is worried about your child?' This may reveal whether or not they admit to a problem with the child, their attitude towards a referring agency and their willingness to accept a diagnosis. Having established these grounds the next question is, 'What is the matter?' It is always better to start from this point and explore, in a thorough and comprehensive manner, the presenting problem and its implications for the child and family before going back to the past history and family history. Sometimes parents will have given their past history so often that it irritates them to recount it, and if it is already catalogued in the notes I find it better just to run through it with them and check on the key points. It is important to remember that contemporary accounts of events are more likely to be accurate than later recall, and engaging in speculation, for example about whether or not it was a very long and difficult labour, is likely to be counter-productive and is best avoided. The aim is to formulate a common understanding with the parents of their child's problem and its implications for them.

Let us assume that all the relevant reports and new developmental assessments are available: can the question 'What is the matter?' now be answered? Usually at this stage a general diagnosis can be given (though a minority of children with undiagnosed developmental delay will remain). Special investigations may already have been performed, but if not this may be a good time to discuss them. For example, should fragile X syndrome be sought in all children with psychomotor delay of obscure origin; in boys only; or in boys with clinical stigmata only? Similarly, there might be discussion about the extra features that would justify performing a CT brain scan, especially if a general anaesthetic is required. It is important to give the parents a balanced account of the issues and to consider their views in addition to assessing the value of the investigation on a cost/benefit basis.

If a diagnosis has been reached by this stage, the question 'What about the future?' can usually be answered in terms of past experience with children with similar problems. Any specific improvements in management which may be anticipated within a reasonable time-scale can be discussed. Often if the diagnosis is general rather than specific, some simple guide to the future can be outlined in terms of likely degrees of dependence, employability, health and survival. The admission of ignorance and of inability to predict outcomes also bears discussion. Sometimes it is necessary to refute suggestions made by the parents about the time-scales of development of particular skills, or even loss of skills, or prognosis for survival in children with neurodegenerative disorders, for instance. It is easy to have words put into one's mouth by parents and often hard to deny that that is happening when the professionally predicted outcome does not coincide with their expectations. Parents often make wishful statements which need correction, and if this is not done they may take their perceptions as confirmed.

More important is the question 'What can be done?'. This is not a question for professionals only. Parents will want to know what they can do, and to leave this question unanswered may lead them to unorthodox practices and 'complementary' medicine. The answer to the question depends on at least two factors: firstly, what is wrong with the child; and secondly, what local facilities are there to help. Conventional therapies are available to most TDCs, and it is generally accepted that early intervention with therapy is beneficial, even if particular proof is often hard to come by (see Chapter 8). For paediatricians, the value of an early intervention programme may be less that it will accelerate the development of psychomotor skills and more that it is something to offer parents which will involve them in a comprehensive support system.

The answer to the question 'What is the cause?' is dependent on how firm a diagnosis has been possible, and care must be exercised here, especially with cerebral palsy, not to confuse cause and effect.

The question 'Will it recur?' is one which can only be answered if the cause rather than the diagnosis is known. Again using the cerebral palsy model, a diagnosis of spastic diplegia in a child born of a blameless pregnancy and delivery will have genetic implications because the cause may be familial. Similar problems are faced in children with severe microcephaly, and rather than exceeding one's brief in this area it is safer to seek the advice of a clinical geneticist.

These are the main questions asked by parents. Beside these, there are other questions from outside agencies to be answered. In the UK, there is a statutory duty to notify Social Service Departments about all disabled children and to notify Education Departments about all children likely to have special educational needs. Further, medical professionals have a statutory obligation to advise parents about the voluntary organisations able to help them. There is often an opportunity at this stage to outline the educational provisions likely to be available for the child, and in the UK the process of 'statementing' for special educational needs should be described if the child is approaching school age.

Style of consultation
Appleton and Minchom (1991) have described models of parent partnership and CDCs. Their observations can be applied to CDCs, TDCs, and individual one-to-one consultations. They suggest four models of parent partnership—the 'expert' model, the 'transplant' model, the 'consumer rights' model and the 'social network/systems' model—and an emergent fifth model, the 'empowerment' model. These are described below.

THE EXPERT MODEL
This is the traditional medical model of work where professionals assess and treat without necessarily making careful reference to parental wishes, views and feelings. There is little negotiation between the parties, and parents may be reluctant to question the professionals' apparent objectives. The approach is mechanistic and has a narrow focus of interest with a lack of fit between parental goals and professional goals.

THE TRANSPLANT MODEL
In the transplant (of expertise) model, parents carry through a particular assessment or treatment programme according to directions given by a professional. Portage services (Cameron 1985, and see Chapter 8), for instance can be regarded as an example of this type of model. Appleton and Minchom list the features of the transplant model as follows:

1   It is assumed that parents know their own children better than any professional can.
2   It is assumed that parents are motivated to help their own children.

3   It is assumed that parents have '24 hour contact' and are therefore in a position to carry through assessment and treatment programmes.
4   It is assumed that the professional will direct the objectives and the method of intervention.
5   It is assumed that the professional will need to be skilled in communication and teaching methods.

This model can be applied not only to intervention but also to the assessment by enabling parents to make relevant observations of the child at home. According to Appleton and Minchom, three problems arise from the assumption that parents can take on the expert role.

1   Differences between families in parenting style and family relationships are not necessarily taken explicitly into consideration.
2   Dependency may be increased because authority and power are seen to remain with the professional.
3   There is a general criticism of both the transplant and the expert model which is evident in recent reports on child health. For instance, Professor Donald Court, as long ago as 1976, commented as follows . .

We are impressed by the way in which the relationship between 'provided services' and the recipients of those services has metamorphosed in the last 200 years of our industrial society. In the beginning the expert and the privileged few tried to provide for the needs of the mass of underprivileged. Then the State began to provide a wider and wider range of services, not only in health but in education and welfare leading to an array of professional organisations, some of which through their sophistication were in danger of alienating those they sought to serve. Professionalism can potentially be a conspiracy against the laity. We believe that in our generation there is the opportunity to make the next essential step and to move to shared responsibility. The laity are no longer the abject poor but the political nation who by their decisions and taxes create and sustain the services they require.

THE CONSUMER RIGHTS MODEL

Various UK governmental edicts in the form of charters, *e.g. The Patients' Charter* (Department of Health 1991), contain strong recommendations about the role of consumers in the control of services. These could be incorporated into the work of the CDC with parents. Appleton and Minchom list the features of this model as follows:

1   It is assumed that parents would have the right to select appropriate services and appropriate interventions for their children. Services would need to provide more information to parents and to provide choices.
2   It would be assumed that parents not only know their own children best, but also know their own current life situation best, and have the expertise to make judgments about the nature of their involvement, as a family, with services.
3   It would be assumed that services need to be highly flexible, not providing standard packages of assessment plus care in specific places, but providing individually tailored help according to parental wishes.

Taken to its fullest extent this model makes the assumption that parents can fully represent their children's and their own needs. To arrive at this point they must be informed of all the services available, and be apprised of their child's perceived needs and prognosis.

They then must be able to select the appropriate services and in partnership with the TDC construct the programme of intervention most suited to the needs of the child and family. This model assumes that there is more time available to the TDC for educating and giving information to each family than is usually the case. Nevertheless, decisions concerning the overall management of a disabled child should be taken in partnership with parents, and the principle is to be encouraged. It should not be overlooked that the child may also have a view here, and the parents, as the consumers of the service, may not always have the child's best interests in mind when they specify the services which they require. For example, they may, unless it is made completely clear, interpret a home-based early intervention programme as a babysitting service. In this model of practice if babysitting or respite care is required, then the parents must be explicit about it.

This model calls for the whole of the TDC service to be managed jointly with parents and for a level of parental choice to select and decide services that is unusual in everyday practice. One can conjure up a picture of families who could operate this model very well and others who would be at a total loss. The latter may be at a loss because they have never been given the responsibility or opportunity to make important decisions concerning their disabled child, but I am confident that there are very many families who could not manage within this model even with extensive support.

There is a further issue that concerns direct or indirect payment for services. In a community where health care is funded from direct taxation and is free at point of delivery, there is a tendency, even a duty, for providers to fit services to needs rather than wants. On the other hand, private patients, *i.e.* those paying directly for itemised services, are in a more powerful position as consumers to specify what they want. Despite the fact that their wants may not correspond to their needs as perceived by professionals, they are more likely to have their way and obtain possibly inappropriate services. In contrast to this, in the expert or transplant models, the patient or family paying directly may be in double jeopardy through having treatments imposed upon them which they may feel to be inappropriate but for which they also have to pay.

THE SOCIAL NETWORK/SYSTEMS MODEL

Here, parents, children and therapists are regarded as part of a network of informal and formal developmental support for the family and child. Of course, this system exists for all children to some extent, and the critical factor is whether the 'professionals' are seen to be part of the family and social network. In this model the social network is recognised and encouraged, with professionals contributing by support as consultants rather than experts, and therapists being regarded as facilitators.

The system is based on a recognition that parents have biographies and that their social circumstances have a bearing on the child's and the family's predicament. Other family members may be a source of support or a distraction in this process of nurturing the disabled child. Thus priorities in helping the family and the target child will be very much modified by the overall ecology.

These factors make an early home visit critical, and the person selected for that responsibility should be the one most likely to have a pivotal role in promoting the child's interests, be it physiotherapist, special education worker or social supporter.

Each person involved with the child in this model has a part in the overall assessment and planning of further services. Each person will have a different perception of the child's needs and priorities. A refocussing on traditional comments such as 'denial', 'noncompliance', and 'difficult families' may lead to different and more constructive commentaries on the predicament of the family and an empowerment for them to redefine their objectives.

THE EMPOWERMENT MODEL

This goes beyond the consumer and social network/systems models. It assumes that parents have control, responsibility and power to make decisions about the child's life. In the context of recognising the strengths of the family and the child, the emphasis is switched to give the TDC responsibility to reorganise and recruit parents into the management team so that parents have a degree of control, not only at family level, but also at various levels in the structure and development of the service. Thus this model would place responsibility on TDCs to:

1   actively promote parents' sense of control over decisions affecting their children,
2   be sensitive to parents' rights to opt into the professional system at a level they choose, and
3   be sensitive to the unique adaptational style that each family and social network will employ.

It is recognised that TDCs, as they evolve and mature, will be able to identify their own styles of working. Traditionally, as more confidence is gained with colleagues and familiarity develops with supporting systems in the community, professionals are able to delegate not only to their trained co-workers but also to parents. Thus there is often an evolution from the expert and transplant models towards the consumer rights, social network/systems and empowerment models. It takes time and confidence to feel at ease working with management committees and steering groups where parents are major participants, and these things need to evolve at a pace which is not necessarily comfortable but is at least measured and controlled.

Having got that far, most people working in this area will recognise that a flexible approach is required and different families require different styles of TDC approach. There will always be those who want the expert model and perhaps they should be empowered or encouraged to do a little more for themselves. On the other hand, there may be some who wish to be empowered not only for their own but for everyone else's family. The style which prevails in the end depends not only on the the experience, personalities and approach of the members of the TDC, but also on the community with its social, economic and political influences. The combinations and permutations are endless, but work from developing countries (Thorburn and Marfo 1990) teaches us that the basis of developmental rehabilitation depends on using the infrastructure (ecology) which already exists and trying to improve it rather than impose a totally new system of intervention on a community which has already evolved its own support structures, no matter how rudimentary.

My own experience in this area is that most parents will seek empowerment if they feel that they are not getting what their children need. We have for many years had parent

representatives on our Portage management group and on our TDC management committee. We ask them to systematically review parental satisfaction or dissatisfaction with the
service provided and contribute to the service planning process, but they need encouragement.

It must be realised that one or two parent representatives may not be equipped or
mandated to set the agenda for all parents. In contrast, however, as Appleton and Minchom
mention, there is considerable dissatisfaction with the special education service because
parents have so little power: our experience is that parents feel much less powerful when
they graduate out of the Portage scheme or out of our local special needs preschool day care
unit (which is run by Barnardos, a UK children and families charity), because parent
representation in the management of the education services is very limited. This has led to
the formation of a group called 'Action Support for the Special Needs Child' which is an
effective lobby supporting the parents' cause through constructive dialogue with the local
education department and organising meetings with talks from interested professionals and
others.

I believe that if parents have the experience of being closely involved in decision
making during their child's early years, it gives them a more positive attitude towards inter-
vening later on when they perceive a service as insufficient.

REFERENCES

Appleton, P.L., Minchom, P.E. (1991) 'Models of parent partnership and child development centres.' *Child: Care,
Health and Development,* **17**, 27–38.
Bax, M.C.O., Whitmore, K. (1985) *District Handicap Teams: Structure, Function and Relationships. Report to
DHSS.* London: Community Paediatric Research Unit, Westminster Children's Hospital.
—— —— (1990) 'Health for all children.' *Archives of Disease in Childhood,* **65**, 141–142. *(Letter.)*
Cameron, S. (1985) 'Parents as educators; learning from Portage.' *In:* De'ath, E., Pugh, G. (Eds.) *Working
Together with Children with Special Needs: Implications for Pre-School Services. Partnership Paper 3.*
London: National Children's Bureau.
Court Report (1976) *Fit for the Future. Report of the Committee on Child Health Services. Vol. 1. Cmnd. 6684.*
London: HMSO.
Cunningham, C.C., Morgan, P.A., McGucken, R.B. (1984) 'Down's syndrome: is dissatisfaction with disclosure
of diagnosis inevitable?' *Developmental Medicine and Child Neurology,* **26**, 33–46.
Department of Health (1991) *The Patients' Charter. Raising the Standards.* London: DoH.
de Winter, M., Balledux M., de Mare, J. (1989) *Early Detection of Developmental Disorders in Young Children.
Results of an International Survey by the Dutch National Committee on Early Detection.* Utrecht Research
Centre on Child Health Care, State University of Utrecht, Faculty of Social Sciences, Netherlands.
Flesch, R. (1948) 'A new readability yardstick.' *Journal of Applied Psychology,* **32**, 221–223.
—— (1949) *The Art of Readable Writing.* New York: Harper & Row.
Hall, D.M.B. (Ed.) (1991) *Health for All Children. A Programme for Child Health Surveillance. The Report of
the Joint Working Party on Child Health Surveillance. 2nd Edn.* Oxford: Oxford University Press.
McConachie, H., Lingham, S., Stiff, B., Holt, K.S. (1988) 'Giving assessment reports to parents.' *Archives of
Disease in Childhood,* **63**, 209–210.
Quine, L., Pahl, J. (1987) 'First diagnosis of severe mental handicap: study of parental reactions.' *Developmental
Medicine and Child Neurology,* **29**, 232–242.
Reed, J., Conneely, J. Gorham, P., Coxhead, S. (1993) 'Assessing the written information given to families prior
to their attendance at a child development centre.' *Child: Care, Health and Development,* **19**, 317–325.
Thorburn M.J., Marfo, K. (Eds.) (1990) *Practical Approaches to Childhood Disability in Developing Countries:
Insights from Experience and Research.* St. Johns, Newfoundland: Project SEREDEC (Memorial University
of Newfoundland); and Spanish Town, Jamaica: 3D Projects.

7
FOLLOW-UP AND FURTHER REFERRALS

An organisation providing services for a local population has a responsibility for ensuring that its attempts to help families in need are monitored. The TDC needs not only to check that services are being delivered but also to establish that they remain appropriate and are modified where necessary.

Children with complex problems may need to be seen regularly in the CDC where the joint expertise of the TDC can be brought to bear. This need not be frequent after the initial problem has been identified and the child's status becomes stable.

Many children having attended the CDC for an initial evaluation can be followed up in other locations. For example, one member of the TDC may attend the child's special school to do clinics there, thus reducing the problem of transport to that of the team member and the parents, as the child has to be at school anyway. Most parents appreciate the opportunity to have their child seen in conjunction with the teacher and therapist at the school. A few prefer to continue attending the CDC because they may be at odds with the education authority or prefer a more 'confidential' setting.

Often appointments with the TDC will need to be phased around appointments in other units, mainly eye, orthopaedic, or ear, nose and throat departments. Planning for follow-up appointments should take this into account. Therefore, planning jointly with the parents helps to minimise the burden of recurring hospital appointments. Parents should always be consulted about follow-ups, because, though the TDC should be aware of appointments with other hospital departments and other agencies, this is not always the case. A single card which incorporates all outstanding appointments is better than a collection of cards from every different department and agency. Some children with epilepsy, congenital heart disease or other acute problems may need to return to the general paediatric clinics between TDC reviews.

What about the children who do not come to appointments? TDC sessions are by nature expensive and missed appointments are costly. If a department experiences frequent defaulting it should first look at its own organisation. Are appointments being sent out in good time, not too far in advance to be forgotten and not at unreasonably short notice? Are they getting to the right address? Does transport need to be arranged? Even if everything is working properly, some disorganised families need reminding with a telephone call, which is after all cheaper than a wasted session of professional time. In a few cases a reminder to the health visitor or equivalent is also required. Some clinics send out a prepaid card which parents return if they intend to keep the appointment: this identifies likely defaulters and allows rescheduling of clinic lists.

What about those who are aware of their appointments but choose not to come? The notes must be reviewed. Do the team's perceptions of the child's needs accord with those of the parents? Has the appointment been made to satisfy the curiosity or other needs of the team rather than the needs of the family? Does the family still have needs which can be met by the team? If the latter is thought to be true then it is probably better to make the next appointment by telephone if possible and obtain confirmation that the family will attend. For recurrent non-attenders a letter should be sent to the general practitioner, with a copy to the parents, explaining that the appointment has been missed and that a further one will be available on request. Sometimes misunderstandings which have arisen between the family and the team can be resolved by using an independent person peripheral to the team who can act as an intermediary and attempt to reconcile the parties involved.

Inevitably in this kind of work tensions and conflicts arise from time to time and these are usually best dealt with by confronting the issues rather than by ignoring them and leaving a child or family 'in limbo'.

Further referrals

An integrated TDC will be able to provide a service which is broader and deeper than the sum of its parts. Nevertheless there will still be some children whose needs cannot be satisfied by their collective expertise. Most teams will have a set of contacts for further referrals. These will depend very much on local geography and professional availability. Ideally one would like to work on a campus where the CDC is adjacent to all the relevant district based services but this is unfortunately a rare occurrence. Some TDCs function by choice in an educational facility which gives them some advantages but excludes readily available specialist medical services. For this reason it may be efficient, and helpful to families, for joint consultations to be arranged in the CDC with various other specialists at infrequent intervals. For example, a child psychologist, if not a core member of the team, might have a monthly session for shared consultations, or an orthopaedic surgeon might be available on a quarterly basis. It may be better to define a clinic by the type of problem it deals with rather than by the professionals practising in it. For example, a mobility clinic would have an orthopaedic surgeon, orthotist and physiotherapist, and not be called an orthopaedic clinic, which implies a single surgical function. Thus these sessions, rather than revolving round a single professional, become specialised TDC clinics. However, that kind of function is more likely to be practicable at regional or tertiary referral levels.

Other children with mainly learning disability will need to be notified to the community learning disability team (CLDT) or its equivalent once they enter their teens, so that plans can be made for their care when they leave school. For this reason and for others, such as the exclusive availability of clinical psychologists or other experts to that team, the TDC should foster good relationships with the CLDT.

Referrals outside district

Secondary referral centres usually do not have more sophisticated services available on site than those described above. Tertiary referral centres or regional centres, using the UK model, are where the more specialised services, such as genetic counselling, neurology, neuroimaging, neurophysiology and gait analysis would be available. Some specialties are more 'portable' than others, and while it may be possible and efficient to get the regional geneticists to conduct combined clinics in the CDC, the laboratory will obviously remain at the centre. Similarly, while the paediatric neurologist should be encouraged to conduct clinics at the secondary referral unit, his or her base will be at the tertiary or regional centre as will most of the investigatory back-up, such as neurophysiology and neuro-radiology. Most neurosurgery in children is performed on an urgent or semi-urgent basis and it is questionable whether paediatric neurosurgical clinics in the CDC are beneficial in terms of improving patient care. The largest group of children involved with neuro-surgeons will be those with hydrocephalus, and the main follow-up and support probably comes from the TDC. The educational and training value of regional consultants visiting the CDCs should carry weight when balancing the pros and cons of such clinics. It is especially important that health service managers should appreciate the training aspect of these specialist visits and not regard them purely in service terms.

With the advent of sophisticated investigation systems such as gait laboratories and advanced cerebral imaging and cerebral function laboratories, there may be greater neces-sity for the child to travel to the regional centre for evaluation. But it also helps greatly with communications if the specialist initiating such investigations sees the child and the family at the local unit before and after the tests are performed. In this way families feel more comfortable with the tertiary referral and with the local team, and the local team becomes more familiar with the systems of investigation and the special techniques involved. This familiarity can often generalise and promote working relationships, understanding and communication between the TDC and the regional unit.

Children are referred to regional units not only for specialised technical investigations but also for the specialised experience and expertise in rare disabilities which can only develop through bringing children with such disabilities into one unit. Different units develop different interests and skill mixes. For example, Rosenbloom's (1990) Liverpool regional unit runs specialised teams for the following: (1) disability register; (2) develop-mental assessment (severe learning difficulties); (3) physical disability; (4) hearing assess-ment; (5) language; (6) visual impairment; (7) behavioural (for children with severe learning difficulties); (8) autism.

These teams have evolved or have been slowly created over a 20 year period. Team membership overlaps considerably, but all have representation from health, education and social services by way of a variety of professional disciplines. The primary functions of each team are: (i) relevant multidisciplinary assessment of relevant children; (ii) descrip-tion and planning of appropriate help; (iii) monitoring the help and the progress that children make; and (iv) promoting the development and availability of relevant resources.

Duplication of assessment, treatment and other resources is avoided as far as possible, not only by the overlapping membership of the various teams but also by ensuring that the most senior staff in all services have a strategic overview.

The full range of services and staffing requirements at regional or tertiary level have been described by Neville (1986).

Requests for second and third opinions
Why is it that parents request second and third opinions more frequently in the area of

childhood disability than in other areas of paediatric practice?

A request for a second opinion in mainline paediatrics, for instance in a child with congenital heart disease or vesico-ureteric reflux, usually comes to the tertiary specialist from paediatricians because they know their limitations in managing the child and are aware of the expertise and facilities available at the tertiary referral centre.

In that case, why does this not happen more often with disabled children, and why do the parents have to make the request? Is it because the paediatricians overestimate their ability to cope with the problem or is it because they underestimate the ability of the tertiary centre to improve on their management? It may be neither. Possibly the paediatrician is correct in thinking that the local team is managing as well as anyone could and there are no other investigations or therapies which would help. Second opinions in children with chronic disability are probably sought more frequently because of the potential scale and duration of the problem. Parents are often still grieving for the child they do not have, and probably have not worked through the well described processes of grief and bereavement (Taylor 1992), in this case losing the wanted and expected child and having a disabled child instead. The sequence of shock, denial, numbness, depression and finally adjustment have to follow. Taylor explored the dynamics of counselling the parents of disabled children and the difficulties of providing them with support. Sloper and Turner (1993) describe the factors that determine the level of parental satisfaction with the disclosure of disability.

This is not to say that grieving does not happen with a child having congenital heart disease, but this can be understood in mechanical terms and usually there is some surgical remedy. With chronic disability, often the underlying cause is obscure, and the prognosis for life and health and education may be imprecise. These two features alone conspire to undermine the parents' confidence in the paediatrician, and if his or her search for answers is unrewarded then they may wish others (both orthodox and complementary practitioners) to take up that task.

I always try to anticipate the request for a second opinion and, if possible, pre-empt it by arranging a joint consultation with the regional paediatric neurologist or other specialist. However, we have all had the experience of parents who seek serial opinions and are difficult to satisfy. Usually they are asking for their own views of the child's problem to be confirmed and will continue to search until someone will do so. Their views can be very entrenched and it has to be appreciated that over the period in which these opinions are sought, the child's problem will have evolved and become clearer as history unfolds. Thus, the best informed opinion is always the most recent one, since the specialist giving it has the advantage of the longest history and the most information. Specialists giving opinions in these circumstances should use their undoubted power responsibly and give the parents realistic expectations not only of their child but also of the services which the local agencies should reasonably be expected to provide. Of course, the commercial market operates here, and there are institutions which, even though some have charitable status, will charge parents considerable sums for the assessment and therapies they offer. To a large extent these institutions have flourished because the orthodox and statutory services for disabled children have been perceived by parents as inadequate, but they may have also been encouraged by professionals who are ignorant of both the local services and the implications for the family of recruitment into a commercial institution or system.

Much has been written about various schools of rehabilitation, and when parents ask about these organisations one has a duty to be frank and open-minded about them. The expectation is that the child will usually come back under local care, and there should be an open door policy for them, and a standing invitation for regular reviews of children who are enrolled on these programmes. If that is not the case, relationships break down, conflicts may arise and the child may suffer, particularly when suddenly presented for school placement having been out of the local system for several years.

Should the request for a second opinion ever be discouraged? One needs to ask, 'For whom am I acting, the parents or the child?' The answer should be both, but sometimes the parents, for their own unreasonable satisfaction, will put the child and its case in jeopardy by hawking it around from centre to centre and specialist to specialist. This does not happen often, but when it does, a long session of counselling with the appropriate team members may bring the process to a halt. In economic terms, repeated opinions are very expensive. It should not be overlooked that a lot of specialist and administrative time is consumed in arranging and executing those consultations. It may be an area where parent-held child health records could come into their own; parents could take their child's record with them to each consultation and if the referral letter is inadequate the notes would be available for further reference. It is certainly daunting to have a thick set of case notes arrive in the post with a brief request for an opinion but no summarising letter from the referring professional.

Who should initiate the request for a second opinion? Should it be the TDC member who usually writes letters, most often the paediatrician, senior clinical medical officer or developmental paediatrician? Should it be the GP, or someone else? Usually it is the person to whom the request is made. If the family asks the GP for a referral elsewhere then the GP should make that referral if s/he agrees that it is reasonable, but s/he does have a duty to notify the people already involved with the family, and sending a copy of the referral letter to the team is the least s/he should do.

If a member of the TDC is asked for a referral, the team can decide with the parents on how that is done and they may recommend that the parents discuss it with their GP before deciding who refers and to whom. Again, everyone involved should be kept informed.

In asking for second opinions it is always helpful to say why this opinion is being sought and who has initiated the process. This gives the referee a good starting point from which to work.

TDC graduates

Many children being followed by the TDC will graduate to adult services. In the UK a well developed system of community learning disability teams (CLDTs) has developed. These will usually have working relationships with the TDC so that children and their parents can be introduced gradually to the appropriate CLDT team members and their support systems. For adolescents with physical disability the situation is less well developed and often there will be no specific person or team to whom referral can be made. These young adults often find themselves consulting orthopaedic surgeons or rheumatologists with no-one over-seeing their total management. As people with normal intellectual development, they have no wish to use the CLDT services and often resent the suggestion that there are therapists within the CLDT who can help them. As Thomas *et al.* (1989) have well illustrated, the needs of these young people are not adequately met in the UK. Similarly, Williams and Bowie (1993) have produced evidence of unmet need in physically disabled adults.

Members of an effective TDC should act as a lobby for their local 'graduate popu-lation' so that their comprehensive care as children can in some way be carried over into their adult life. Each team will need to consider local circumstances, assess needs and make recommendations to the appropriate authorities.

An effective TDC will develop ways of using registers (see Chapter 10) to keep the information concerning each child under its care up-dated and relevant. The consultant paediatrician in community child health or equivalent is the best final pathway for this information which the TDC will pass on to school doctors and medical staff in health clinics. Similarly there will be a flow of information from other agencies such as education and social services. There should always be opportunities for discussion of children with complex problems between the various agencies, and any individual should be able to call a case conference empowered to activate such a discussion in the same way as one is for child protection procedures. Bradford (1993) describes how multi-agency consultation teams can establish effective inter-agency collaboration in complex cases.

The TDC does not need to follow up all the children it sees, and many can be dis-charged back to the primary health care team. Communications at this stage are important, especially if therapies are to continue. Not only is medical information vital, but other TDC members should communicate, independently if necessary, with their counterparts in the community. A letter summarising any residual problems and giving advice on general man-agement, on the child's strengths and on potential problem areas, is mandatory. The offer of some sort of re-referral if problems arise later gives the primary care team confidence that the child is not being abandoned.

REFERENCES

Bradford, R. (1993) 'Promoting inter-agency collaboration in child services.' *Child: Care, Health and Develop-ment*, **19**, 355–367.
Neville, B.G.R. (1986) *Services for Chronic Disability in Childhood and Adolescence in the United Kingdom.* *BPA/BPNA Working Party Report to the DHSS.*
Rosenbloom, L. (1990) 'Multi-disciplinary assessment: hope versus experience.' *Paper presented to the 2nd Meeting of the European Academy of Childhood Disability, Durham.*
Sloper, P., Turner, S. (1993) 'Determinants of parental satisfaction with disclosure of disability.' *Developmental Medicine and Child Neurology*, **35**, 816–825.
Taylor, D.C. (1982) 'Counselling the parents of handicapped children.' *British Medical Journal*, **284**, 1027–1028.
Thomas, A.P. Bax, M.C.O., Smyth, D.P.L. (1989) *The Health and Social Needs of Young Adults with Physical Disabilities. Clinics in Developmental Medicine No. 106.* London: Mac Keith Press.
Williams, M.H., Bowie, C. (1993) 'Evidence of unmet need in the care of severely disabled adults.' *British Med-ical Journal*, **306**, 95–98.

8
THERAPIES AND OTHER INTERVENTIONS

What do parents want?

Before discussing what therapies are available and the scientific or other justification for recommending them, it is useful to consider what parents feel they need.

In her book *The Costs of Caring,* Sally Baldwin (1985) asked parents of disabled children what would be the most useful form of help for them at the present. She found that more of them (31 per cent) mentioned financial help than any particular service, but that twice as many gave priority to some other service (Table 8.1). Better medical services appeared to be a very low priority; however, the TDC can also promote some of the other services which Baldwin has listed. Her book contains many quotations from parents, and considers ideas concerning the balance between giving needy families cash allowances so that they can buy-in services, and having those services provided by the supporting authorities. In-depth interviews revealed that substituting cash allowances for services in kind was attractive, with the majority of parents preferring to be given an adequate amount of money to spend as they see fit 'without red tape or interference'. They expressed a strong desire to minimise the frequency with which they had to be assessed for help, principally by local agencies and particularly through assessments which involved 'means tests'. Further, Beresford (1993) reports the effect of financial support from government funds administered through an independent organisation (the Joseph Rowntree Foundation) and given to families with a disabled child. It was found to reduce the mother's perception of the stresses of caring for the child and improve her sense of well-being and adjustment.

When we see children and their families in clinics we are usually unaware of their financial position even if we know the family quite well and have a note of the parents' occupations. It is worth bearing in mind the findings recorded above when considering the priorities we may have for the child and family, as compared with the family's own priorities. We can then go on to consider in which of the areas where help is most needed we can be most influential.

When the family has had it confirmed that the child requires some intervention process, be it because of learning problems, motor disorder or challenging behaviour, the question the parents ask is what can they do to help. Indeed, as a rule they are the individuals most motivated to help. Another dimension to this is the stress on the family that results from the disability of the child and what can be done to relieve it. Rosenbaum *et al.* (1992) have attempted to examine the factors which cause stress to the parents of physically disabled children and to identify the components of care giving as judged by both professionals and parents to be important in minimising this. From questionnaires sent to professionals involved in the management of physically disabled children in Ontario, they generated a priority list of the important components of care (Table 8.2). Similar responses and priority lists were obtained from the parents of these children (Table 8.3).

TABLE 8.1
Responses of parents of disabled children to the question,
'What help would you find most useful at present?'

	N	%
More financial help	105	} 31
Financial help with transport	43	
Someone to look after the child sometimes to give us a rest	90	19
Better education and training facilities	80	17
Better housing	54	11
Someone to give advice, information and encouragement	44	9
Better facilities for long-term care	30	6
Better aids and equipment	19	4
Better medical services	12	3
Cannot say	3	—
Total	480	100

Reproduced by permission from Baldwin (1985).

TABLE 8.2
Professionals' ranking of 22 components of care
(percentage of respondents selecting components
of care in top six of 22)

	%
Treatment of disability	75.9
Evaluation of disability	70.4
Team approach	60.2
Parental involvement	54.0
Accessible/available	45.5
Co-ordination	44.3
Education/information	43.2
Continuity and consistency	31.0
Emotional support	29.9
Family-centred approach	28.7
Diagnosis	27.6
Advice on development	24.1
Facilities	22.7
Anticipatory guidance	19.5
Home and community outreach	14.9
Non-professional social support	4.6
Support for professionals	4.6
Future planning	1.1
Genetic counselling	1.1
Advocacy	0
Acute illness care	0
Well-child care	0

Adapted by permission from Rosenbaum *et al.* (1992).

TABLE 8.3
Parents' ranking of 22 components of care
(percentage of respondents selecting components
of care in top six of 22)

	%
Parental involvement	61.4
Education/information	57.8
Treatment of disability	50.0
Accessible/available	49.0
Continuity and consistency	37.1
Co-ordination	36.8
Family-centred approach	35.9
Evaluation of disability	32.7
Diagnosis	32.5
Facilities	30.9
Advice on development	28.9
Non-professional social support	25.9
Advocacy	25.6
Emotional support	24.6
Team approach	18.3
Home and community outreach	14.9
Anticipatory guidance	14.2
Future planning	11.3
Acute illness care	8.3
Support for professionals	6.5
Genetic counselling	4.9
Well-child care	2.5

Adapted by permission from Rosenbaum *et al.* (1992).

The results indicated that although 'team approach' was important for the professionals, who ranked it third out of 22, for the parents (who ranked it 15th) it was considerably less important. It must be remembered that the parents surveyed belonged to parent support groups and presumably understood the importance attached by professionals to team work.

In contrast, parents ranked parental involvement first by a clear margin, whereas professionals put it fourth, making it less important than treatment of disability, evaluation of disability and team approach. In their additional free comments parents most frequently cited respite services as a major requirement in addition to the listed components of care. We should therefore not assume that our traditional approach and attitudes about therapies and interventions match precisely what parents feel they need, especially where stress reduction is a major consideration.

O'Sullivan *et al.* (1992) conducted a study to obtain information about parental satisfaction with paediatricians across the broad spectrum of services that have been recommended for disabled children and their families. The sample comprised 503 mothers (from the middle socioeconomic group) of children below seven years of age with developmental disabilities. The results indicated that the mothers found paediatricians quite informative about their children's medical conditions and helpful in assisting them to obtain other relevant medical resources. However, there was a lack of paediatric involvement in family centred issues despite the call (in USA Public Law 99-457) for physicians to take a more expansive role in providing care for disabled children and their families. O'Sullivan *et al.* went on to discuss training in this area and the lack of financial reward for physicians practising in family centred services and concluded that both factors may be inhibiting the commitment of physicians to the psychosocial concerns of families of young disabled children.

Traditional therapies

As demands on therapists increase and recruitment into training becomes more difficult, the concept of the therapist as teacher of therapy to carers rather than as a 'hands on' therapist becomes stronger. Traditionally what parents expect of a physiotherapist is a certain period of time working with the child each day. That is logistically impossible in this context, but for therapies to be effective they have to be be carried out for a defined length of time at defined frequencies (Bower and McLellan 1992). In most societies this is possible only if the parents do the 'hands on' work. Therefore therapists must be able to explain the rationale for the intervention, demonstrate it, teach it to parents and carers, and re-evaluate and modify it as necessary.

Occasional home visits by therapists, especially at the onset of therapy, are important. The physical layout of the home and the available facilities will determine to a large extent what is possible for the parents or carers to achieve. This is mandatory for occupational therapists where problems of access, mobility within the home and outside, and possible modification to the home need to be addressed. Often the occupational therapist responsible for such domestic aids and modifications may be responsible to a different agency from the physiotherapist. In the UK the social services departments have occupational therapists with this remit, whereas the physiotherapists and occupational therapists who advise on activities of daily living are health authority employees. Again the need for communication between the TDC members and other agencies is crucial.

Therapy in the home carried out by the parent or carer under the periodic supervision of the therapist appears to be the main avenue for delivery of physiotherapy, but what about speech therapy? Speech therapists or speech and language pathologists have a rather more entrenched tradition of working directly with children rather than through parents or carers. However, shortfall in recruitment in this area is forcing therapists to change their style and they too are now increasingly working through parents and carers.

Thus we come to the concept of parents and carers as therapists. It is a concept that is fundamental to intensive intervention programmes such as that prescribed by the Doman and Delacato Institutes and their various related schools (Doman 1974) and the Portage early intervention programme (Shearer and Shearer 1976). Systems not working through parents, such as Conductive Education, depend on the availability of extensively trained conductors who also assume a part of the parental role. Harnessing parental enthusiasm to work with the child and giving them the expertise to do so is an important part of the responsibilities of the TDC. In turn the power given to the parents by promoting their interests and giving them proper status can be channelled into management, and into the political system to influence the provision of services for their children.

Therapists do not necessarily need to work in a one-to-one system. There are occasions when it is helpful to get together a group of children with similar disabilities, and their parents, and for the therapist to teach general principles of therapy and then look at the few specific problems which may be more or less common to the group. This style promotes parental involvement with other parents and allows them to realise that there are other children with similar problems which may respond to similar or different interventions. In other circumstances the therapists may work with the children and nursery teachers, or just the children in a group. Palmer *et al.* (1988), in a large trial, demonstrated that for diplegic children, routine use of physical therapy had no short term advantage over infant stimulation. Experience and experimentation will help decide how to use the therapist's resources most efficiently and effectively. Constant evaluation and audit of systems employed, as well as audit of outcome, will promote this.

Physiotherapy
Scrutton (1984) in the introduction to his book *Management of the Motor Disorders of Children with Cerebral Palsy*, pointed out that there are many variables within each type of cerebral palsy, and that family and other circumstances complicate the therapy requirements. 'Doctors can choose to ignore these complexities simply by referring the child for 'therapy'; therapists cannot.' His book contains a chapter on neurodevelopmental treatment by Karel and Berta Bobath which gives a comprehensive view of their philosophy and techniques. The Bobaths maintain that eclectic treatment, using a mixture of treatments and treatment techniques derived from various schools of thought which see the child's problems from different viewpoints, cannot result in a cohesive programme. Nevertheless, one suspects that most physiotherapists do not practice pure Bobath or a pure discipline of any

school unless they are constrained within the parent institution. Conductive Education is referred to below, but again is well outlined in Scrutton's monograph by Hari and Tillemans.

My own feeling is that while recognising that schools of physiotherapy have their disciples there is more faith and belief controlling their loyalty than there is science and logic. Until some better rationale for intervention is described and superior techniques to improve function are devised, I am inclined to support the Aim Orientated Management proposals of Scrutton. He describes the dilemma: firstly, whether to treat, and secondly, what to treat. His focus is on management and aims, and he states that experience points to the conclusion that the effective parts of treatment are those which become part of the child's life. When this happens, a comparatively small (but carefully selected) therapy input has a significant effect. The management must extend into the child's family and school environment. He gives concrete examples of Aim Orientated Management, stating that they are subservient to one overriding aim: an endeavour to guide the children towards adulthood with a purpose in life and with the best possibility of fulfilling themselves.

Further practical points of therapy management for cerebral palsy are given by Green (1992) and Jones *et al.* (1992). Finnie (1974) has written for parents of children with cerebral palsy, and therapists would do well to know what is being recommended directly to the parents of their patients in publications of this sort.

Speech and language therapy
The role of the speech and language therapist is probably rather broader than that of the physiotherapist in that a larger spectrum of disorders is covered. These range from children with neuromotor problems specifically involving the apparatus of feeding and articulation through the various types of language disorder to children with the autistic syndromes. Thus the whole range of disorders, from physical to psychiatric, including perhaps the purely emotional categories, may be subjects for the speech and language therapist.

The most frequently encountered disorder of speech and language development is that of children with global developmental delay who are usually a little further behind in their language skills than in other areas. The demands of parents for therapy for these children when their needs are probably of a more general nature saps the limited resources of speech and language therapists who might be more effectively engaged with children who have specific language problems. This is an area where a general intervention programme might be a more cost effective way of delivering the service and Portage (see below) can achieve this. The development of teams of therapists and medical officers to consider such children and prioritise their needs should help.

At a tertiary referral level, speech and language therapists have a major role to play in the organisation of intervention programmes involving alternative or augmented forms of communication for language impaired children (Jolleff *et al.* 1992). A good example of joint work between speech and language therapists and other professionals on a supra-regional basis is that of the Consortium on Drooling (Blasco and Allaire 1992). It is from study groups such as this, which survey sufficient patients and experiences of intervention to make valid recommendations for management, that we will best learn how to deal with what have hitherto been regarded as intractable problems.

Occupational therapy

In the UK, occupational therapists are much in evidence in departments caring for the elderly and in adult rehabilitation centres. In children's units they are not so well represented. It may be that mobility and gross motor problems have exercised those caring for children disproportionately. The day to day activities of small children are looked after by their parents, and the fact that disabled children may require rather different handling and help to cope with these activities is easily overlooked. This is where the occupational therapist may be able to promote children's abilities to cope for themselves with a reduction in parental intervention. Sadly it is often only when the child assumes adult physical proportions that the burden for parents becomes too great and only then that the services of an occupational therapist are sought. Help at this stage often takes the form of initiating modifications to the architecture of the home and introducing aids for lifting and mobility. In the UK such intervention is managed through the social services departments whereas the hospital and community based occupational therapists would be employed by the health authority. One would like to see a more comprehensive occupational therapy service which considered all aspects of the child's activities of daily living, following the child and his or her family from the CDC to the home and providing advice, practical support and interventions over the long term. Then interventions could be properly planned and not initiated only in crisis as is so often the case now.

In the early years the occupational therapist can advise Portage workers, as the physiotherapists and speech and language therapists do, with the Portage worker being the final common pathway to the family, rather as the Conductor is the final common pathway to the child in Conductive Education.

Other interventions

Early intervention programmes for children with psychomotor problems have become established in many countries during the last decade, and their effectiveness has been questioned (Sylva 1989). To begin with there was a belief that these programmes would ameliorate children's disabilities and give them a higher IQ than would otherwise have been the case. An overview has recently been provided by the Infant Health and Development Program (1990). In his commentary on this meta-analysis, Richmond (1990) stated that this was the largest study of a comprehensively enriched programme for preterm low birthweight infants and it had demonstrated significant improvement in cognitive and behavioural function over the first three years of life. He pointed out that there was as yet no evidence that the improvement is sustained beyond three years of age. He also underlined the importance of identifying groups that may benefit the most from intervention programmes, noting that very low birthweight babies with IQ scores below 70 seem to be less likely to improve than others. He commented significantly that family circumstances such as levels of parental education and economic status are important indicators as to which children are most in need of intervention.

Barrera and Rosenbaum (1992) drew attention to the work of White-Traut and Nelson

79

(1988) in finding that maternally administered physical stimulation to preterm infants in the nursery resulted in improvements in mother–infant interactions prior to hospital discharge, but the sample was mostly of disadvantaged mothers. The same did not hold for a sample of white middle-class mothers (Booth *et al.* 1985). White-Traut and Nelson's findings could be considered as a description of 'taking up the slack' in deprived and potentially deprived children. Barrera and Rosenbaum went on to comment:

Considering these studies combined, we can conclude that supportive intervention for parents of their low birthweight premature infants during the first year of life results in significant benefits for both children and parents. These benefits are likely to diminish the risks of cognitive delays, school failures, and behavior and socio-emotional disturbances often found in this population. Moreover, supportive intervention is likely to promote positive parent-child interactions as part of the overall improvement of developmental outcomes, which in turn may result in a lower burden of suffering for these families.

The question remains as to whether skills and IQ achieved are ultimately better than would have happened without help or whether they will be gained at a faster rate with an ultimate outcome no different from that which would have occurred naturally. These arguments in my view are not very relevant. Most parents want to help their children attain their best potential and that is why they ask for our help.

There are many different ways of helping, and choosing the best for an individual child used to be very difficult. Before any early intervention programmes were available, we used to attempt to describe to parents what their child's weaknesses and strengths were and give a brief account of how best the child could be helped. For the clinicians, this was not only very time consuming but put unrealistic demands on their knowledge and experience of the therapies available. Parents consequently became frustrated and looked elsewhere for help. Often this would result in their recruitment onto programmes where the demands on the family and child were inordinate and the results not commensurate with the efforts expended.

Meisels and Shonkoff (1990) in their *Handbook of Early Childhood Intervention* have produced a masterly and comprehensive review of all aspects of early childhood intervention. Much of it is rather theoretical and academic for the general clinician or therapist, but it does provide a firm scientific basis for the processes, and for the evaluation of results. In the preface to their book they quote the passing of the Education for All Handicapped Children Act Amendments of 1986 (USA Public Law 99-457) as giving early intervention a growing national importance, increased funding, a promise of more comprehensive programmes and services, and unprecedented attention for major state and federal policy making groups. They proffered a general definition:

Early childhood intervention consists of multidisciplinary services provided for developmentally vulnerable or disabled children from birth to age 3 years and their families. These programs are designed to enhance child development, minimize potential delays, remediate existing problems, prevent further deterioration, limit the acquisition of additional handicapping conditions, and/or promote adaptive family functioning. The goals of early intervention are accomplished by providing developmental and therapeutic services for children, and support and instruction for their families.

Unfortunately in the UK neither the Warnock Report (1978) nor the Children Act of 1989 impinge significantly on this area of need. The legislation is open to liberal interpretation, and the discretion given to local authorities contrasts with the statutory obligation in the USA for provision of early intervention.

What follows are comments on some of the main early intervention programmes in use today.

Portage

Portage is named after the town in Wisconsin where the programme was first developed in 1969 by Shearer and Shearer (Shearer and Shearer 1976). For Portage workers the title is something of a disadvantage since they have to explain it to everyone newly introduced to it. The programme was introduced in the UK in research projects in 1978 and as a service programme from 1980. Over 200 Portage projects started during the following decade and continue today. It has also been introduced to many other developed and developing countries (Thorburn and Marfo 1990). Sturmey *et al.* (1992) have recently reviewed cross-cultural aspects and intra-cultural variability of Portage, and Arvio *et al.* (1993) have demonstrated an impressive internal consistency and reliability of the assessment scale. They also found good cross-validation against the traditional tests of mental development including the Stanford–Binet, WISC-R, WPPSI, Merrill–Palmer, Bayley, Leiter and WAIS.

The basis of the programme is that the intervention is delivered at home by the parents with usually weekly supervision by the Portage visitor. One of the best firsthand accounts of the Portage model has been given by Jesien (1984). He discussed the history, described the method in detail and speculated on the reasons for its success.

Programmes have been set up by various agencies including health, education, social services and voluntary organisations. It is probably most efficient for the primary and secondary health care teams to initiate referrals into the programmes since they are the people most likely to have first contact with young children who have developmental problems. Some children having an obvious physical marker of developmental risk, such as Down syndrome or spina bifida, can be expected to require the service from an early age, but others can be introduced when their need is perceived. Health visitors and their equivalents have an important role to play here in introducing these children to the service.

Local criteria need to be set for admission to the programme. They should include: degree of disability of the child; geographic catchment area; number of families to be served at any one time; age of the child; availability of other services; and willingness of parents to participate.

The Portage system is relatively prescriptive, and gives parents a well described task to accomplish with the child and a formula for recording success and failure. This means it is very unusual to find parents who are intellectually incapable of administering the programme. However, a few parents do not have the motivation, while, in contrast, some have expectations which are so unrealistically high that they are unable to limit themselves to the prescribed tasks and ask too much of the child.

The goals must be set jointly by the Portage adviser and the parents. A weekly visit is the norm. All goals targeted, achieved or failed are recorded, and a cumulative check-list of achievement is compiled. Criteria for graduating out of Portage also need to be set.

Programmes should be administered by a local management group with parent representation. Some programmes have voluntary Portage advisers, some of whom are parents who have had a child on the programme and have subsequently themselves undergone the necessary training course as a home adviser.

The benefits resulting from Portage are not only an acceleration in acquisition of skills (a benefit we have observed in two thirds of the children in our unpublished series, and especially in those from deprived environments), but it also offers support to the family and provides a link between them and the other statutory and voluntary services. Our own programme has generated a parents' group who compile a regular newsletter and directory of families on the programme. They also help with fund raising and publicity. An audio tape describing the programme has been sent to every local general practitioner, and video tapes have been prepared for fund raising purposes. One recent innovation is to have parents video their children carrying out the programme at home and for the tape to be viewed at the next TDC consultation. The whole exercise is steered by the Portage management group which comprises members of the TDC together with the Portage supervisor, representatives from the local education department, and parent representatives.

Using trained Portage visitors with varying backgrounds—*e.g.* health visitors, therapists, teachers, parents—results in a higher level of competence than if they were all from one discipline. They have weekly or bi-weekly joint meetings, often with other therapists or psychologists, to give general or specific help with particular case problems. The parents also invite therapists and others to their group meetings.

In this way, families become familiar with all the services available, are able to identify what is not available but needed, and can act as a pressure group to highlight and remedy shortcomings in services. They also generate a spirit of camaraderie and mutual support.

Portage, along with any other early intervention programme, needs to be viewed in the context of any other available local service, such as special nursery school provision for preschool children with learning problems, and other self-help groups.

There is, of course, no panacea for children with developmental disorders, and to promote a programme so as to give that impression to parents, either consciously or unconsciously, is wrong. Portage is labour intensive for advisers and for parents. Some parents may feel guilty that they do not allocate adequate time to the programme, although this might apply to any intervention using parents as the therapeutic vehicle.

Another problem can be to make the child and parents too dependent upon one-to-one activities, but as long as the adviser is aware that this is a potential problem it can be avoided by engaging the family in other group activities.

The key issue is organisation of the programme, keeping the team motivated and ensuring a quality service. This requires an enthusiastic, self-perpetuating team with readily available help from psychologists, therapists and management, and periodic retraining. If regular meetings and periodic retraining do not happen, the programme will fail.

From the responses (unpublished) to questionnaires which we sent to all the families who had been on our project over a ten year period, we found that even when parents of profoundly disabled children had not perceived gains in ability in the child as a result of the programme, they would still recommend Portage to other families because of the general support which it provides. In a section for free comments, parents additionally indicated that they wanted to have feedback on their own performance. They generally can see how well the child is doing: they need to know how well they are doing themselves.

Doman–Delacato
Doman and Delacato established the Institutes for the Achievement of Human Potential in Philadelphia in the 1960s. Their work was described comprehensively by Doman (1974). Their exacting technique of recruiting cohorts of helpers to carry out intensive pro-gramming exercises with disabled children has been widely criticised (Cummins 1988). However, the important effect they had on mainstream paediatric practice was to stimulate paediatricians and therapists into devising ways of answering the familiar question from parents, 'How can I best help my child develop?' The result of this is the recognition that early intervention programmes are needed and that if parents cannot get help locally they will go to where it is available, irrespective, in some cases, of distance and personal cost. Several services have evolved in the UK and elsewhere based on the Doman and Delacato techniques but employing programmes which are less demanding on parents.

Conductive Education
The Peto Institute in Budapest has received a great deal of attention in recent years. Their process, Conductive Education (CE) (Hari and Akos 1971, Hari and Tillemans 1984), is quite different in concept and delivery from the Doman–Delacato method. Pepper (personal communication) visited both Philadelphia and Budapest and summarised the different approaches as a product of the different political and social systems in the two countries. The Doman–Delacato method, in a free enterprise culture, holds parents and their own self-recruited helpers responsible if targets are missed, whether through inad-equate effort or inappropriate goals. The CE system smacked of a state-run enterprise with third parties (the conductors) taking over the parental role in a sophisticated kind of social welfare system. A number of other paediatricians and professionals visiting Budapest have produced reports of mixed feelings about the system (Beach 1988, Robinson *et al.* 1989). Essentially, CE depends on the holistic skills and approach of the conductors, who are trained in education and therapy in a relatively long and exacting course. In this scheme the parents are rather excluded. One of the main criticisms is that the children admitted to CE are highly selected (Bairstow *et al.* 1991) and would be likely to do well under most rehabilitation programmes (Bax 1991). Despite the apparent view (Sutton 1988) that real CE can only exist in Hungary, it has been evaluated at The Foundation for Conductive Education Unit in Birmingham, UK (which is funded by the Department of Health). The full evaluation has now been published (Bairstow and Hur 1993), and the evidence that CE has great benefits over orthodox treatment is lacking. However, the report has been severely criticised by The Spastics Society (Hancock 1993) for not evaluating CE as a system. Bax (1993) reviews the findings and suggests that not many people are objectively measuring outcomes in this field. He encourages advancement on a broader front to

develop effective means of helping the child with cerebral palsy.

In the UK there are several institutions practising a modified form of CE and other units where different therapies and philosophies, *e.g.* reflexology, are used.

Parents who attend these units often identify features of them which could be more generally employed. They feel they are treated as valued clients; the venue is usually comfortable and not 'clinical'; the staff are said to be friendly and non-judgemental; and the child is assessed and treated on a very personal basis. Generally parents are impressed by this approach and it would not be too difficult for us to incorporate the main features into our own routine practice. Interestingly, parents often share my scepticism about the validity of reports produced by some of these organisations, detailing improvements their systems have achieved. Most feel, however, that they are getting a service, though some are disillusioned.

Specialised day nurseries

The provision of specialised day nursery places for special needs children is very patchy in the UK and at the mercy of local authority education departments who do not always perceive this provision as having high priority. In some other European countries and the USA the provision appears to be rather better. There is no doubt that in addition to individual work, special needs preschool children also need opportunities to socialise with their peers, and this is what nurseries provide. It is important that these provisions are seen as therapeutic or educational and not as a baby-sitting service. The needs of the children, particularly in the area of language development, should be met with adequate provision of speech therapy advice, physiotherapy for those requiring it, and good staff ratios. In addition to therapy these placements can facilitate invaluable observations of the child's abilities and relationships in 'free range', rather than in the formal testing situations in which some children under-perform.

Because places in special nurseries are at such a premium, good organisation and management is required to oversee the financial aspects and prioritise children for admission on the basis of their needs, the interventions available, and the likely benefits. This is an exacting task and requires multi-professional involvement with representation from the local TDC.

Toy library

There are many variations in the way toy libraries work. In the UK, the National Toy Libraries Association is a charitable trust and most local toy libraries are affiliated to it. Toy libraries may be mobile, perhaps in a large bus visiting needy residential areas. Some are associated with a unit at the Portage scheme's base, with Portage workers selecting toys for the child and delivering them, or with children and parents coming to the library to choose. Similarly, the CDC may have a toy library or it may be attached to the special needs nursery. The main function of the toy library is to provide children with a source of play material appropriate to their developmental age and to give them extra enjoyment. It should not, in my view, be seen as overtly promoting education. Children need fun and to be able, as far as possible, to select what materials they require for this. A further value of the toy library is to provide a meeting place for parents, especially if that is not available elsewhere. Social and informal contacts can be set up, and by having regular hours of opening a critical mass of parents can be got together to meet. This group may decide to organise other functions such as picnics, outings and lectures.

Similarly, soft play areas, again very expensive to construct, act as a focus for parents and children using the facility; sited within CDCs, they help provide fun and relaxation in daily life. Local nursery children can get to know disabled children and the CDC if they are allowed to use the soft play area jointly from time to time. This may promote knowledge and acceptance of disability in preschool groups at a time when more integration of disabled children into mainstream schools is already happening.

Parents groups and special interest groups

Whether they have guidance and encouragement from 'professionals' or not, parents will get together and form groups. Some individuals are socially outgoing and some less so, and not all will want to be involved in groups. Some of the most effective parent interest groups are those which have informed officers who are respected by the professionals with whom they work. These groups may be set up initially by the professionals who should then take a back seat and be available in an advisory capacity once a group has 'taken off'.

Groups come in many forms, local and national, general and specialist. Professionals can learn a lot about rare syndromes from the publications produced by some of the specialist parent groups who often are aware of contemporary research developments before they reach generalist journals. In the UK there is a legal requirement for parents of special needs children to be put in touch with the appropriate voluntary organisation for their child. Local groups may grow up around an early intervention programme or around the CDC. They need to be given direction initially but can then run their own affairs and provide representation for, *e.g.* the Portage management team or TDC management group. Without parental representatives on these groups there is no way of incorporating user views into the management system. Our local Portage parents' group produces a regular newsletter and directory of Portage parents.

Some of the parents of special needs children attending the specialised Barnados nursery have gone on to form a group called Action Support for the Special Needs Child. They are a well informed group who are familiar with legislation regarding health, social services and education, and are powerful in promoting the needs of their own children and of special needs children in general. Among other activities, this group advises and supports parents whose children are undergoing the statutory process known as statementing for special educational needs. They can act as advocates for the children and parents and give them the power to question professional decisions on a confident, informed basis.

Such powerful self-help groups have managed in our location to persuade the social services department to re-open residential respite care places which had been closed on financial grounds.

Working with these organisations and giving advice only when required, rather than gratuitously, is rewarding, especially since they are often a useful source of advice to the professionals.

These groups tend to wax and wane according to the ages of their children and the leadership within them, but we should always be ready to encourage and help in their constructive efforts.

Evaluation

As more intervention programmes are initiated and therapies introduced, there is an increasing need to establish criteria for measuring efficiency and value for money. Some attempts to do this have been made (Berry and Wood 1981, Shonkoff *et al.* 1988, Hauser-Cram 1990). It behoves us all to make some attempt to establish the value of the services we provide by whatever means we can. Certainly justification of labour intensive intervention programmes is likely to become a more pressing requirement of health and education service funders.

REFERENCES

Arvio, M., Hautamäki, J., Tiilikka, P. (1993) 'Reliability and validity of the Portage assessment scale for clinical studies of mentally handicapped populations.' *Child: Care, Health and Development,* **19**, 89–98.

Bairstow, P., Cochrane, R., Rusk, I. (1991) 'Selection of children with cerebral palsy for Conductive Education and the characteristics of children judged suitable and unsuitable.' *Developmental Medicine and Child Neurology*, **33**, 984–992.

—— Hur, J. (1993) *Evaluation of Conductive Education for Children with Cerebral Palsy. Final Report (Parts I and II).* London: HMSO.

Baldwin, S. (1985) *The Costs of Caring. Families with Disabled Children.* London: Routledge & Kegan Paul.

Barrera, M.E., Rosenbaum, P.L. (1992) 'Supporting parents and promoting attachment'. *In:* Sinclair, J.C., Bracken, M.B. (Eds.) *Effective Care of the Newborn Infant.* Oxford: Oxford University Press, pp. 221–246.

Bax, MCO. (1991) 'Conductive Education.' *Developmental Medicine and Child Neurology*, **33**, 941–942.

—— (1993) 'Conductive Education assessed.' *Developmental Medicine and Child Neurology*, **35**, 659–660. *(Editorial.)*

Beach, R.C. (1988) 'Conductive Education for motor disorders: new hope or false hope?' *Archives of Disease in Childhood*, **63**, 211–213.

Beresford, B.A. (1993) ' Easing the strain: assessing the impact of a Family Fund grant on mothers caring for a severely disabled child.' *Child: Care, Health and Development*, **19**, 369–378.

Berry, I., Wood, J. (1981) 'The evaluation of parent intervention with young handicapped children.' *Behavioural Psychotherapy*, **9**, 358–368.

Blasco, P.A., Allaire, J.H., and participants of the Consortium on Drooling (1992) 'Drooling in the developmentally disabled: management practices and recommendations.' *Developmental Medicine and Child Neurology*, **34**, 849–862.

Bobath, K., Bobath, B. (1984) 'The neuro-developmental treatment.' *In:* Scrutton, D. (Ed.) *Management of the Motor Disorders of Children with Cerebral Palsy. Clinics in Developmental Medicine No. 90.* London: S.I.M.P., pp. 6–18.

Booth, C.L., Johnson-Crowley, N., Barnard, K.E. (1985) 'Infant massage and exercise: worth the effort?' *Maternal Child Nursing Journal*, **10**, 184–189.

Bower, E., McLellan, D.L. (1992) 'Effect of increased exposure to physiotherapy on skill acquisition of children with cerebral palsy.' *Developmental Medicine and Child Neurology*, **34**, 25–39.

Cummins, R.A. (1988) *The Neurologically Impaired Child. Doman–Delacato Techniques Reappraised.* London: Croom Helm.

Doman, G. (1974) *What To Do About Your Brain Injured Child.* New York: Doubleday.

Finnie, N.R. (1974) *Handling the Young Cerebral Palsied Child at Home. 2nd Edn.* London: Heinemann.

Green, E.M. (1992) 'Cerebral palsy: postural stabilisation.' *In:* McCarthy, G.T. (Ed.) *Physical Disability in Childhood. An Interdisciplinary Approach to Management.* Edinburgh: Churchill Livingstone, pp. 159–162.

Hancock, R. (1993) *Conductive Education - Research Report.* London: The Spastics Society. *(Letter addressed to parents.)*

Hari, M., Akos, K. (1971, translated 1988 by N. Horton Smith and J. Stevens) *Conductive Education.* London: Routledge.

—— Tillemans, T. (1984) 'Conductive education.' *In:* Scrutton, D. (Ed.) *Management of the Motor Disorders of Children with Cerebral Palsy. Clinics in Developmental Medicine No. 90.* London: Spastics International Medical Publications, pp. 19–35.

Hauser-Cram, P. (1990) 'Designing meaningful evaluations of early intervention services.' *In:* Meisels, S.J. Shonkoff, J.P. (Eds.) *Handbook of Early Childhood Intervention.* Cambridge: Cambridge University Press.

Infant Health and Development Program (1990) 'Enhancing the outcomes of low-birth-weight, premature infants. A multisite, randomized trial.' *Journal of the American Medical Association*, **263**, 3035–3043.

Jesien, G. (1984) 'Home-based early intervention: a description of the Portage project model.' *In:* Scrutton, D. (Ed.) *Management of the Motor Disorders of Children with Cerebral Palsy. Clinics in Developmental Medicine No 90.* London: S.I.M.P., pp. 36–48.

Jolleff, N., McConachie, N., Winyard, S., Jones, S., Wisbeach, A., Clayton, C. (1992) 'Communication aids for children: procedures and problems.' *Developmental Medicine and Child Neurology*, **34**, 719–730.

Jones, M., Moffatt, V., Mulcahy, C.M., Nicholls, C.S., McCarthy, G.T. (1992) 'Cerebral palsy: therapy management.' *In:* McCarthy, G.T. (Ed.) *Physical Disability in Childhood. An Interdisciplinary Approach to Management.* Edinburgh: Churchill Livingstone, pp. 115–157.

Meisels, S.J., Shonkoff, J.P. (Eds.) (1990) *Handbook of Early Childhood Intervention.* Cambridge: Cambridge University Press.

O'Sullivan, P., Mahoney, G., Robinson, C. (1992) 'Perceptions of paediatricians' helpfulness: a national study of mothers of young disabled children.' *Developmental Medicine and Child Neurology*, **34**, 1064–1071.

Palmer, F.B., Shapiro, B.K., Wachtel, R.C., Allen, M.C., Hiller, J.E., Harryman, S.E., Mosher, B.S., Meinert, C.L., Capute, A.J. (1988) 'The effects of physical therapy on cerebral palsy: a controlled trial in infants with spastic diplegia.' *New England Journal of Medicine*, **318**, 803–808.

Richmond, J. (1990) 'Low birth-weight infants. Can we enhance their development?' *Journal of the American Medical Association*, **263**, 3069–3070.

Robinson, R.O., McCarthy, G.T., Little, T.M. (1989) 'Conductive education at the Peto Institute, Budapest.' *British Medical Journal*, **299**, 1145–1149.

Rosenbaum, P.L., King, S.M., Cadman, D.T. (1992) 'Measuring processes of care giving to physically disabled children and their families. I: Identifying relevant components of care.' *Developmental Medicine and Child Neurology*, **34**, 103–114.

Scrutton, D. (Ed.) (1984) *Management of the Motor Disorders of Children with Cerebral Palsy. Clinics in Developmental Medicine No. 90.* London: S.I.M.P.

Shearer, D., Shearer, M.S. (1976) 'The Portage project: a model for early childhood intervention.' *In:* Tjossem, T.D. (Ed.) Intervention Strategies for High Risk Infants and Young Children. Baltimore: University Park Press, pp. 335–350.

Shonkoff, J.P., Hauser-Cram, P., Krauss, M.W., Upshur, C.C. (1988) 'Early Intervention efficacy research: what have we learned and where do we go from here?' *Topics in Early Childhood Special Education*, **8**, 81–93.

Sylva, K. (1989) 'Does early intervention 'work'?' *Archives of Disease in Childhood*, **64**, 1103–1104.

Sturmey, P., Thorburn, M.J., Brown, J.M., Reed, J., Kaur, J., King, G. (1992) 'Portage guide to early intervention: cross-cultural aspects and intra-cultural variability.' *Child: Care, Health and Development*, **18**, 377–394.

Sutton, A. (1988) 'Conductive education.' *Archives of Disease in Childhood*, **63**, 214–217.

Thorburn M.J., Marfo, K. (Eds.) (1990) *Practical Approaches to Childhood Disability in Developing Countries. Insights from Experience and Research.* St. Johns, Newfoundland: Project SEREDEC (Memorial University of Newfoundland); and Spanish Town, Jamaica: 3D Projects.

Warnock Report (1978) *Special Educational Needs. Report of the Committee of Enquiry into the Education of Handicapped Children and Adults. Cmnd 7212.* London: HMSO.

White-Traut, R., Nelson, M. (1988) 'Maternally administered tactile, auditory, visual and vestibular stimulation: relationship to later interactions between mothers and preterm infants.' *Research Nursing Health*, **11**, 31–39.

9
EDUCATION

Educating the team

Any organisation, if it is to grow and develop, should adopt a policy of being open to criticism and should be able to evaluate its own objectives and achievements. In this setting, it is possible to change direction, to learn from the change and to evaluate its effects. This process is known to some as clinical audit and is an exercise in education and development.

Members of a team have a responsibility to themselves to be well informed in their own area of expertise and to keep up with developments. They also need to be aware of the training curriculum and ethos of their colleagues from different professions. The effects of differing educational and perceptual outlooks are well described by Lyon (1988). She looks at the differences in orientation toward the concept of learning disabilities in various professional groups, and compares the perceptions of paediatricians and teachers. She finds that paediatricians refer to psychological evaluation, family history and teacher's reports, whereas the teachers put more faith in 'medical techniques', for example physical and neurological examination. Paediatricians are aware of the inconclusiveness of their investigations, whereas teachers expect a more exact medical diagnosis.

The rate of increase in knowledge in different disciplines varies. In particular, the range of medical investigatory techniques has increased dramatically in the last few years in comparison with the steady but slower progress in educational theory and practice. Thus team members of different disciplines have a responsibility to each other to appraise colleagues of advances in their fields of activity which are relevant to the work of the team. This kind of interchange, together with discussion of other advances which are not directly applicable but are of general interest, reinforces team spirit and identity.

Funds should be available to allow team members to attend courses and training programmes which will develop their professional effectiveness. Members should be willing to report back, either in writing or by presenting highlights of the course, to other team members and other members of their professional group. Training is even more valuable for teams when two or three team members attend meetings, together with members from other services, so that experience of team dynamics as well as professional function can be shared. The true transdisciplinary team will welcome this kind of exercise but logistically it is the most difficult to arrange. In some institutions, granting study leave for such events would be made conditional on some process of reporting back.

Ensuring that there are adequate financial and other resources for the fundamental requirement of training the team is a key responsibility of management. Of course it is cheaper in the short run not to supply a service than to do so, and cost conscious managers cannot be expected to initiate new services of any kind. The motivation must come from the team.

Joint work with tertiary centres

A natural development of education for TDCs would be to use their links with regional or tertiary referral centres and to engage visiting consultants from the centres in formal as well as informal teaching sessions. This can be done on the days of their visits, though it needs careful planning: the clinical load for such visitors is often very heavy, and it is unfair to burden them further with a large formal teaching commitment.

The tertiary centre itself should organise educational activities to keep the district personnel up-to-date with services offered and types of referral to be encouraged. It should also be involved in some kind of quality control process highlighting good practice in the districts and helping those with shortcomings to remedy their service shortfall. When this process is channelled through educational activities it is less likely to be construed as critical than if weaknesses are baldly stated in management reports—though those who fail to respond to the gentle pressure of peer review may require more persuasion.

The primary care team

In addition to its own education, the TDC has a responsibility for the education of other groups. In this context, the primary care team of general practitioner and health visitor can be considered as one unit and the TDC needs to be willing to involve itself in their continuing education. Health visitors or their equivalents are often the main source of input to the TDC and they must be kept informed of the team's activities and services with frequently updated material.

Audio or video tape can be used effectively as a teaching method: for example, the existence, availability, entry criteria and basic functions of an early intervention programme, such as Portage, can be detailed on audio or video tape and sent to local primary care teams. Drug companies, for instance, have found using audio tapes effective for promoting their products: they know that GPs spend many short periods of time in their cars and will listen to promotional material whereas they often ignore or overlook written material.

Other opportunities for informing GPs are available at postgraduate education meetings, especially in the UK where a financial allowance from the health authority encourages GPs to attend a certain number of such sessions each year. TDCs should also target their local Vocational Training Scheme for general practice and make it conditional that if members of the team are required to teach these trainee GPs to become accredited in child development surveillance, the trainees should also be made aware of the further diagnostic services and interventions available for children who are referred as having special needs through this system. Thus the young GPs are given the skills required by the trainers and the additional knowledge they will need in their future relationship with the TDC.

Students and junior staff

Training medical students and junior staff poses a particular problem for the TDC. One system has been well described by Rosenbloom and Marlow (1990). They outline four initial precepts. First, trainees must be aware of the balance between investigational, diagnostic and therapeutic paediatric medicine on the one hand, and family relationships, children's needs and parental adjustment on the other. They must also recognise the gulf between ideal and practical provision of community and other support services. Secondly they must appreciate that disabled children and their parents relish continuity of care with a doctor with whom they have an established relationship. Thirdly, the trainee should be aware that the main contributions to the management of disabled children are normally made by people other than doctors; and lastly, that care for such children only rarely takes place within the hospital.

They go on to describe the content of their training programme and how it is incorporated in the sequential procedures that families follow when children are referred.

Evered *et al.* (1989) have described a system for the training of senior registrars in child psychiatry by employing them to carry out liaison psychiatry in a CDC. This is an important training issue and ties in well with the concepts described by Sturge (1989) (see Chapter 4). Both papers underline the importance of the relationship between child psychiatry and CDCs and describe the strategies and tactics of working together, giving useful models for service provision and training.

Parents

Team members have much to learn from both general and specialised parent groups and have an obligation to involve themselves in both informal and formal educational transactions with them. These activities take place at many levels ranging from a few explanatory words at a consultation to conducting joint research projects. There are many opportunities between these two extremes to exchange information using, for example, printed material, audio tapes and video tapes.

Producing a handbook for families of special needs children is one example of good practice. Such a handbook should give details of the statutory and voluntary services available for special needs children, both at national and local level. Each handbook will be unique: we have found it best to divide ours into preschool, school and post-school sections. Handbooks quickly become out of date, particularly if the names of helpers, rather than titles, are given, and a regular update is essential. Compiling such a handbook is a useful exercise for TDC members for their own education and because it often reveals shortcomings in local services (see Appendix 2, pp. 105–107).

Ferlie *et al.* (1984) considered a 'helping booklet' when evaluating joint working in the care of mentally handicapped people. They found problems with layout, content and distribution. Subsequently, however, when studying the same groups three years later, these workers found that distribution of the booklet had improved, that 80 per cent of recipients found it useful, and that there was a greater degree of satisfaction with information amongst parents in a health authority which had a booklet compared with one which did not (Quine and Pahl 1989). With careful planning, the problems of layout, content and distribution can be avoided. Smith (1992) informs us that writing simple English is difficult even for doctors, and Albert and Chadwick (1992) describe some general practice leaflets and find that many GPs are extremely concerned with the technical aspects of such leaflets, for example the quality of printing, photographs and illustrations. Yet some clearly ignore or misunderstand the needs of their readers, and a minority neglect the straightforward (and comparatively cheap) techniques of good, simple, common communications. Albert and Chadwick explain the use of the 'Gunning fog' test of readability and use it to compare practice leaflets for readability with other forms of writing such as novels, newspapers and insurance policies. These principles of simplicity and clarity should be applied to any publication where popular readership by lay people is the aim.

Some TDCs will encourage parents to use a common professional/parents library in the child development centre and others will develop an information service specifically for parents, such as a 'special needs information centre'. A centre of this type will contain a computerised database with an index of literature produced by relevant statutory bodies and by various charitable groups and self-help organisations. In the UK, the *Contact a Family (CaF) Directory* (1991) would be a key reference tool for such a centre.

Each centre would have a range of literature such as that referenced by Donovan *et al.* (1989) in their paper concerned with the need for and use of written educational material by the parents of 41 children with cerebral palsy. Many of these parents had attempted to find suitable literature but only two thirds succeeded.

Both parents and professionals should be encouraged to use the database and help to expand the pool of information by sending new material to the key organiser. Such a centre can be run on a voluntary basis if a few interested professionals have the motivation to initiate it.

This kind of centre enables parents to combine an information gathering exercise with social support and increases their contacts with other families and professionals and their confidence in dealing with their own disabled child.

The newsletters and journals of specialist groups are of great value in bringing the hard information that is first published in research papers to the attention of parents and interested professionals, before it is covered by more generalist journals. A recent article in *RTMDC News*, the magazine of the Research Trust for Metabolic Diseases in Children, entitled 'Lowe's syndrome – the gene is found!' (Fig. 9.1) is a good example of this. The article was widely distributed to members of the research trust and interested professionals. It drew attention to the announcement in the July 1992 issue of *Nature* concerning the isolation and identification of the gene causing Lowe syndrome in a straightforward and effective way. Blake and Brown (1993) have described how a parent support group was able to provide information concerning a specific syndrome (CHARGE) which helped to delineate the syndrome, the associated defects and possible aetiology—again illustrating how parent groups can contribute to doctors' knowledge, as well as *vice versa*.

The general public
There are two main reasons for educating the general public about children with special needs. The first is that society should be aware of its less privileged members and be encouraged to take some responsibility within the community for at least recognising, and at best promoting the needs of less privileged citizens. A planning application for a sheltered home for half a dozen children with learning difficulties in the neighbourhood would be resisted less by those who understand the implications than by those who do not.

Planning, of course, comes into most aspects of community life and includes con-

HQ News

Lowe's Syndrome –
The Gene is Found!

Researchers announced in the July 16 issue of *Nature* that they have isolated and identified the gene that causes Lowe's syndrome, a rare hereditary condition that causes physical and mental handicaps and serious medical problems. The discovery was the result of a 7 year research project partially funded by the Lowe's Syndrome Association Inc., USA.

Lowe's (oculo-cerebro-renal) syndrome is an x-linked inherited disorder that affects males. Females may be carriers of the gene and pass it on to their sons. Features of the condition include congenital cataracts, glaucoma, weak muscles, mental retardation, kidney problems, short stature, seizures, behaviour problems, bone problems, and shortened lifespan. Physicians estimate there are about 200-400 cases of Lowe's syndrome in the United States.

Until now the exact locations and identity of the gene that causes Lowe's syndrome was unknown. The discovery of the gene is "the biggest research breakthrough since the syndrome was first recognised 40 years ago," according to Kaye McSpadden, Medical Research Chair of the Lowe's Syndrome Association (LSA).

Leaders of the research team, Robert L. Nussbaum, M.D., of the University of Pennsylvania School of Medicine, and Richard A. Lewis, M.D., of Baylor College of Medicine in Houston, reported that they have been able to determine the genetic code of a major portion of the Lowe's syndrome gene. Their research also strongly suggests that the Lowe's syndrome gene controls the production of a specific enzyme, inositol-polyphosphate-5-phosphatase.

As a result of these findings, families will soon have more help available to them in the area of genetic counselling, including a reliable and relatively simple test to determine who is a carrier of the gene. Also, the enzyme discovery will open the door to further investigations into the under-lying metabolic defect and how it leads to the various medical problems. New and more effective methods of treatment may develop as a result. Dr. Nussbaum said, however, "This is just the beginning. Much more work needs to be done."

Kaye McSpadden, who founded the LSA in 1983, said, "This discovery is our dream finally beginning to come true. When our son was diagnosed 14 years ago they told us no one was interested in doing research because the condition was rare. Part of the reason we started the LSA was to change that. Now, we can look into the future with real hope and know that we made a difference."

Dr. Lewis, a member of the LSA's Scientific Advisory Committee, said the research project would not have been possible without the participation of the 78 families whose genetic histories were studied and whose members gave blood samples and underwent eye examinations.

The LSA is an international non-profit organisation made up of about 350 parents, professionals, and others who are interested in the condition. The purposes of the organisation are to foster communication and mutual support among families, provide information, and support and encourage research. Two research grants from the organisation provided partial funding for the gene research project.

From the LSA Press Release – July 16th, 1992.

Fig. 9.1. Specialist groups are often the first to bring new findings to the attention of parents and professionals. (Reset from the original article in *RTMDC News*, by permission.)

siderations of wheelchair access and services for visually and hearing impaired persons. Again, attitudes would be more tolerant were public awareness of disabilities enhanced.

The second reason for the TDC having a high public profile is for fund raising purposes. Given the current levels of public expenditure in this area, the team whose members can identify and target charitable organisations and organise direct fund raising exercises will have much more flexibility in its service delivery. It will become less constrained by the financial stringencies imposed on statutory bodies and may be able to afford the extra initiatives which make all the difference between an adequate service and a special one. Services for disabled or special needs children are a relatively emotive area, and with enthusiasm and flair considerable funds can be raised even from communities not known for their wealth and affluence.

That is not to say, of course, that the statutory organisations should not be held responsible for what they are legally bound to provide, and there are good examples of joint working between charitable organisations and the statutory bodies. For example, the Barnardos charity in the UK runs a number of special needs day care nurseries in co-operation with local education and social services departments and subsidises them generously.

Facilities

Specific facilities are required for educational activities, and the well equipped CDC will have a room for meetings, with appropriate audiovisual equipment. This will often double as the case conferences room. A library in the building is essential, and the relevant journals and reference books for both professionals and parents should be available. It is best to involve the local medical librarian in ordering, cataloguing and displaying books and periodicals. This avoids duplication and helps the librarian run an integrated service. Photocopying facilities close to the library reduce the loss of journals and periodicals and encourage the dissemination of information. It must be emphasised to management that these facilities are essentials, not luxuries, and as such should be part of the normal budget for the centre or team.

REFERENCES

Albert, T., Chadwick, S. (1992) 'How readable are practice leaflets?' *British Medical Journal*, **305**, 1266–1268.
Blake, K.D., Brown, D. (1993) 'CHARGE association looking at the future - the voice of a family support group.' *Child: Care, Health and Development*, **19**, 395–409.
Contact a Family (1991) *CaF Directory of Specific Conditions and Rare Syndromes in Children, with their Family Support Network.* London: CaF.
Donovan, T.J., Reddihough, D.S., Court, J.M., Doyle, L.W. (1989) 'Health literature for parents of children with cerebral palsy.' *Developmental Medicine and Child Neurology*, **31**, 489–493.
Evered, C.J., Hill, P.D., Hall, D.M., Hollins, S.C. (1989) 'Liaison psychiatry in a child development clinic.' *Archives of Disease in Childhood*, **64**, 754–758.
Ferlie, E., Pahl, J., Quine, L. (1984) 'Professional collaboration in services for mentally handicapped people.' *Journal of Social Policy*, **13**, 185–202.
Lyon, C.S. (1988) 'Comprehensive medical evaluation of children with learning disabilities: comparison of paediatricians' and teachers' perceptions.' *Journal of Learning Disabilities*, **13**, 19–24.
Quine, L., Pahl, J. (1989) *Stress and Coping in Families Caring for a Child with Severe Mental Handicap: a Longitudinal Study.* Canterbury: Institute of Social and Applied Psychology and Centre for Health Services Studies, University of Kent.
Rosenbloom, L., Marlow, N. (1990) 'Teaching junior staff about caring for handicapped children.' *Archives of Disease in Childhood*, **65**, 903–905.
RTMDC News (1992) 'Lowe's syndrome–the gene is found!' *RTMDC News*, **4**(3), 4. *(Editorial.)*
Smith, T. (1992) 'Information for patients—writing simple English is difficult even for doctors.' *British Medical Journal*, **305**, 1242.
Sturge, J.C. (1989) 'Joint work in paediatrics: a child psychiatry perspective.' *Archives of Disease in Childhood*, **64**, 155–158.

10
LIAISON

Notes

The medical notes of children with long-standing complex disability are often bulky, disordered and frustrating to deal with, especially if the user is unfamiliar with the child or the note-keeping system. For a child with, for example, cerebral palsy, epilepsy, learning problems and sensory problems, many different medical specialists and therapists will have data to enter into the notes and information which they will need to retrieve later.

How can we best keep the bulk and weight of these records to a minimum while preserving the quality of the content?

Every new initiative in management appears to generate its own avalanche of documentation. This makes it essential that superfluous paperwork must be weeded out and discarded if relevant data are to be preserved effectively. For instance, our special care baby unit recently changed its computerised note-keeping system so that now each baby in the intensive therapy unit has a sheet generated daily by the computer which details all the care provided during that day. At the end of the week the seven daily sheets are summarised on to one sheet. Previously, the daily sheets and the seven-day summary were all being filed and the notes became bulky and unmanageable: not a good start, when an end of stay summary could potentially replace 100 or so sheets with two or three.

The problem with notes is that everyone wants his or her own special element, inevitably giving rise to reduplication. When I see children with complex problems for the first time, I attempt to write a summarising letter which incorporates all the relevant past history and will act as a basis for further communications. This needs to be headed up with diagnosis where available and problems or symptoms where the diagnosis does not incorporate those aspects. This must be done in such a way as to make use of the International Coding of Disease and Symptoms, or other coding system, possible.

Other issues hinge on the number of sets of notes needed for each child. Does the TDC need to have its own notes separate from other medical notes? There is no doubt that one set of notes for each child is by far the best arrangement. It would be very frustrating if the CDC or TDC had notes separate from those of the orthopaedic department and psychiatric department. And yet this happens. Furthermore there are few health authorities where the notes of the community child health service and hospital service are unified, but that is what we should aim for. If a child has only one set of notes it is much less likely that complicating factors will be overlooked and that data will be mislaid. For example, if relevant data are entered into common notes, much letter writing between professionals might be avoided. It is also easier to organise clinic appointments which do not clash if one knows when the next ophthalmology or orthopaedic consultation is due. Similarly, it is easier to identify missed appointments with specialists who do not send reminders after failed appointments. Psychiatrists often want to keep separate notes but this risks keeping other professionals in ignorance not only of the extent, but also of the fact of their involvement with a particular child or family.

Ongoing notes

Ideally, the initial summarising statement concerning a child with complex problems should be capable of periodic updating. If traditional notes are kept, regular rewriting is required. When word processing or computer facilities are available it is possible to develop a system whereby the initial summarising statement can be updated without total revision. For instance, past history and family history (using dates of birth rather than ages) can be preserved and later information modified. This requires a structure where it is recognised that certain parts of the communication will be stable over time and certain parts variable. Such data can be kept manually by using a structured history sheet that fulfils its function in much the same way that problem orientated medical records list inactive and active problems (Weed 1968). The process can be applied to all children attending the TDC or to only those with complex problems, the others being adequately dealt with in the traditional way. If computer systems are to be used, then it is most likely that a common system will be employed for all children.

It is surprising how often basic information of the 'can do' and 'can't do' type is left out of medical notes. Possibly we get too close to the patients, concentrating on recording the detail and failing to record the obvious: not recording, for example, the mode of mobility, but then being unable to recall it from memory when asked about it. For this reason, professionals often prefer a structured kind of note-keeping, so that an *aide-mémoire* or check list is incorporated into the system ensuring that every aspect of the child's repertoire is considered on each occasion.

This may be too prescriptive. The menu for the consultation should be generated for each child at the pre-clinic planning phase (see Chapter 6) and there should not be a blanket interrogation on each occasion. Different people use notes differently, some as a form of shorthand from which to generate structured reports, others as a detailed commentary in the form of an essay on the consultation.

Each of us has our own style, but we should not forget the purpose of notes, which is to record facts, opinions, and transactions and plans for the future in a form making it possible to recall information easily and, if necessary, to transmit it accurately to others.

With our own interests in note-keeping we often overlook the needs of others among whom there are two principal groups: parents and planners.

Notes and parents

Should parents hold the notes of their children? There is no doubt that note-holding by patients can be effective, and in obstetric practice it is becoming accepted that pregnant women carry their own medical notes. It is also accepted that the child health record of growth, immunisation status and general data should be held by the parents of every child. At present, however, it is not practicable for parents to be the caretakers of the notes of a child with complex problems. They may often be used as their couriers from department to department, however, and Jolly (1984) recommended that patients or parents should keep

TABLE 10.1
Parents' comments on the usefulness of written reports

Category	Frequency (N = 25)
Jogs memory—too anxious at the time to take all in	11
Can look back and read again in the future and see progress made	8
Can 'mull over' what has been said	5
Can discuss with husband and family	5
Can discuss with professionals	5
Outside view, from a different angle helps you to stand back and pin-point areas where child needs help	5

Reproduced by permission from McConachie *et al.* (1988).

their own notes. Further, in his unit, a letter was compiled embodying the findings of all members of the child development team together with an agreed plan of management. This was sent by post to parents and a copy, together with the technical reports of each professional, was sent to the GP. Parents could then go to their GP to discuss elements of the letter which required clarification. However, for parents to have the only copy of the collective notes would make it very difficult for professionals to communicate about a child since for most of the time they would not have access to the notes.

Partridge (1984) described a system where reports were compiled specifically for parents and discussed how content is altered for the lay consumer. The key worker appeared to be the final editor, and s/he was required to deliver the report to the parents and then to comment on their reactions to it. In his survey, out of the 133 occasions when reports were compiled, 98 of 115 parents were satisfied with such reports, seven needed further explanation, 11 had some moderate difficulty, nine found the written reports upsetting and eight parents found them very useful. The point was made that written reports provide a useful addition to the assessment process but cannot replace face to face consultation and counselling.

McConachie *et al.* (1988) reported on the reactions of 25 parents to receiving copies of written reports concerning the developmental assessment of their children (Table 10.1). In this case parents received the same report as was sent to the professionals. Reports were popular with parents of older children—*i.e.* those who may have had longer to think about and accept the nature of their child's disability—tending to be more positive. Either technical terms were explained in the body of the report or parents were encouraged to discuss them, and the whole report, with the relevant professionals. Suitably presented, numerical results could be sent to parents without raising alarm.

Giving parents certain summarising information concerning their child is now regarded as good practice. This may be in the form of a report generated specifically for them after an assessment procedure. However, this implies that there is another, different report for professionals and thus the clerical activity is doubled. Alternatively, the parents can be given a copy of the 'common report' which is written in language which can be understood by lay persons. It is much better to appear to one's professional colleagues to be over-simplifying than to baffle parents with cryptic medical jargon. After all, in the UK medical notes generated after November 1991 are by law accessible on request to the patient or his or her agents, so there is no reason in general for not being open. Additionally, parents become very frustrated by being repeatedly required to give a detailed history to every professional they meet. This is particularly significant where families move from district to district and arrive to see new professionals before the notes or correspondence from their old ones have got there. The ownership of a comprehensive report gives them a little more power and confidence at a new consultation than might otherwise be the case.

Notes and planning

Notes and the information contained in them can be used for planning purposes only if the information is readily accessible. In order to study work load, activity levels and diagnostic groups and to gather data suitable for planning the service, a great deal is demanded of case notes. Summarising data—including name, date of birth, address, diagnostic group, functional analysis of disability, interventions required, interventions anticipated, and responsible education authority and social services authority—are fairly basic elements. If computers are to be used, these elements must be capable of being coded. It is clear that a common data base between the community child health service, the hospital service, and the education and social services is very desirable. Both social services and education authorities need to know about special needs children from the moment their needs are first recognised. For planning purposes the data can be made anonymous, and for epidemiological inter-district comparisons and audit purposes this anonymity must be assured.

Registers

Colver and Robinson (1989) have described how to establish a register of children with special needs. Their objectives were: (i) to improve the care of the individual children; (ii) to improve the planning of services for children; and (iii) to improve opportunities for research and epidemiology.

The Court Report (1976) recommended the keeping of such registers by each health authority. Colver and Robinson's register (of children in the Northumberland health district) includes: (a) children with chronic illness; (b) children subject to a statement of special educational needs; and (c) preschool children who already need special educational provision or help from many professionals. The register does not include: children with congenital malformations (which in the UK are already on the Office of Population, Censuses and Surveys Register), most of whom do not give rise to long term special needs; children 'at risk of a condition', a concept now largely abandoned; or children with common mild chronic conditions, *e.g.* asthma or glue ear, unless the condition by its severity or complex interaction with family factors creates a long term special need, in which case, such a child is registered on the basis of the special need, not on the basis of the medical diagnosis.

Colver and Robinson recognise grey areas such as a child with a mild hemiplegia or one requiring remedial help with reading, and a consistent approach to these 'marginal' cases is required. They write:

TABLE 10.2
Data recorded for each child on computer register of
children with long term special needs in Northumberland
health district, UK

Unique computer number
Surname
First name
Address
Date of birth
Sex
County district
Family doctor
School
School doctor
Free text description of child's main diagnoses
Coding of above diagnosis
Coding of impairment
Coding of disability
Medical provision—for example, paediatrician
Educational provision—for example, preschool teacher
Therapeutic provision—for example, physiotherapist
Family provision—for example, attendance allowance
Date of educational statement

Reproduced by permission from Colver and Robinson (1989).

'Diagnosis' is not a logical system of classification for it may describe a disease, medical problem, impairment, or psychological circumstance. Nevertheless the concept is very useful and we have developed a 100 category classification relevant to children with chronic problems. Each child may have up to six codes. For instance a child with Down's syndrome may be coded as Down's, fostered, complex heart disease, mental retardation, glue ear.

The concepts of impairment, disability, and handicap are more logical and consistent but the World Health Organisation coding system is complex. Moreover, it was not designed for children and does not take account of age or the effects of handicap on the family. We have recorded data about impairment and disability as one research objective on the register.

The information recorded for each child by Colver and Robinson is listed in Table 10.2. Input is by a medically qualified practitioner from data supplied by neonatal units, hospital discharge summaries, outpatient letters, health visitors and the local education authority. To keep the register up to date a list is sent every year to each school doctor to confirm or change the school which a child attends. Also, when an examination is under-taken for the 1981 Education Act the doctor completes a form for the computer data base.

Colver and Robinson make the point that each district must establish the validity of its register before it can be used for planning, research or epidemiology.

They produce figures for their own system which show that:

. . for more severe impairments our register is as, or more, comprehensive than external lists. For less severe impairments such as diabetes we are not so comprehensive. . . For preschool children there are few independent data sets with which to compare a register. We suggest as a measure of validity the

TABLE 10.3

Examples of uses to which the Northumberland register of special needs children is put.

Individual care

The names of preschool children are brought up for review by the preschool panel for children with special needs. One function of this panel is to inform the education department of preschool children likely to have special educational needs

Preschool children with certain problems are notified to the community dental service

Information is sent to each school doctor about children with special needs in ordinary and special schools

Planning

Information to the principal educational psychologist enabled him to apply successfully to the Department of Education and Science for funds for a 'Portage scheme'

Information to a specialist health visitor and social worker helped them assess the need for and subsequently introduce a parents' support group for families with disabled children

Information to the social services department helped them plan further developments in their respite care service for families with disabled children

Information to the Spina Bifida Association enabled it to plan voluntary services in Northumberland

Research and epidemiology

Evaluation of the health surveillance programme of preschool children in Northumberland requires regular details of children with congenital deafness, severe cerebral palsy, language delay and mental retardation

A regional study of cerebral palsy received information about children with cerebral palsy

Three separate national studies of congenital rubella, autism and deaf–blind children received information about such children

The Family Fund in York compared its register with the Northumberland register and reported the proportion of children with severe disabilities who applied to the fund

A working party of the British Paediatric Association received a report on the prevalence of disabling conditions in childhood in Northumberland

Adapted by permission from Colver and Robinson (1989).

number of children, unknown to the register while preschool, who became subject of an educational statement before age 6 years.

They record five such children in the previous three years from a population of 290,000. The point is made that the register must 'live'. The more it is used, 'the more accurate and comprehensive it becomes.' They provide examples of uses to which their register is put, as reproduced in Table 10.3.

They make the comment that little attention has been paid to the objectives, criteria for registration or validity of registers held by health districts, and observe that if the small amount of data on each child is kept up to date, confidence will grow and opportunities for individual care, service planning, research and epidemiology will improve. Finally, they suggest that the uses to which a register is put 'must be regularly reported to the staff who contribute data so that the relevance of the register is appreciated and its accuracy thereby maintained.'

Woodroffe and Abra (1991) have also described a special conditions register (SCR). The data base in West Sussex in the UK was set up in 1971 and initially developed around

TABLE 10.4
Variables recorded in child health system from birth notification (West Sussex Area Health Authority)

- Mother's age and obstetric history, including exposure to risk factors (for example, smoking, X-rays) and use of medication during pregnancy
- Perinatal details, including mode of delivery, birthweight and gestation, Apgar score, postnatal jaundice, convulsions, or respiratory distress
- Birth order
- Congenital malformations
- Family history of illness—*e.g.* tuberculosis, Down syndrome, haemophilia
- Socioeconomic group

Reproduced by permission from Woodroffe and Alba (1991).

TABLE 10.5
Variables recorded in the West Sussex special conditions register

- Main functional disability: physical, developmental (<5 years), educational (≥5 years), sensory vision, sensory hearing, speech, psychological, multiple
- Disability severity; none or mild (not requiring special treatment or schooling, early stages of chronic disease—*e.g.* Still's disease, cystic fibrosis, diabetes mellitus), moderate (needing treatment or special schooling—*e.g.* moderate learning difficulties, developmental delay with developmental quotient <70), significant (needing special schooling or increased support), or severe
- Diagnosis by ICD9 and supplementary codes
- School or unit attended
- Use of aids—for example, wheelchair or hearing aid
- Year of statement of special educational need

Reproduced by permission from Woodroffe and Abra (1991).

the central file on all children for the purposes of 'immunisation and vaccination, early child health, school health, and special conditions'.

The file is initiated by the birth notification (Table 10.4), results of neonatal screening for phenylketonuria and hypothyroidism, immunisation status, and the results of scheduled 'screening' throughout childhood as reported by the laboratory, health visitor, GP, clinical medical officer, school doctor or school nurse. Information recorded in the SCR is listed in Table 10.5.

All the health and education professionals involved with the child at any point send reports to the system. There is a 'constant unscheduled updating' of the SCR in addition to a manual scheduled updating:

Each health visitor receives a list of children under 5 years of age in her practice whose names are on the SCR, to check their entry, and to identify children who should be added to or removed from the list. For school age children a list is sent for checking to each school doctor and nurse.

The uses of the SCR include the 'opportunistic review of individual cases by the community paediatrician' who is responsible for maintaining the system. It is also used to ensure that the local education authority has been notified by the age of two years that a child may have special educational needs, and that the social services department is provided with the register of disabled children required under the Children Act 1989.

Examples of recent use of the SCR include identifying the number of children with hearing aids, the number of visually impaired children in mainstream school, and the number of children under five years with developmental problems who will require nursery places. Once such a register is established and its data validated (by, for example, as in this system, comparing the SCR's record of diabetic children living in the area with other local records), there is a whole range of epidemiology and outcome information available. Woodroffe and Abra comment that, while the accuracy of the data increases with the number of sources of information, conversely 'accuracy has been found to decrease with the number of variables recorded for each child, and most importantly with the mobility of the child population. Although the SCR is updated until age 19 for children who remain in school, accuracy declines after age 16 when register entries for children who have left school are no longer reviewed each year by the school medical officer, and incident cases age 16–19 may never be added to the SCR.' The SCR is maintained primarily for the care of individual children and for planning services. For the care of the individual child, addition to the register is more important than deletion. For planning services the priority is an up to date list of resident prevalent cases and their future service requirements. For aetiology, the priority may be an accurate list of all incident cases in the birth cohort and their history of exposure. Local and national priorities also conflict.

Clearly there is a need for compatibility between registers and, as Woodroffe and Abra plead, a national policy for health information systems for children with special needs. Without this the potential contribution to continuity of care for individual children, to planning and monitoring services at regional and national level, and to facilitating research in the aetiology and treatment of uncommon conditions will be lost.

As the registers described above confirm, the technology is available, but input must be by a competent medical officer and regular updating and validation is vital. A national system incorporating a minimum database is required which can be expanded and enhanced according to local requirements. Only in this way will it be possible to scrutinise, for instance, the outcome data of babies of birthweight <1000g looked after in 'regional units' compared with those looked after in 'other units', or to audit the effectiveness of the hearing distraction tests performed by health visitors and make district to district comparisons.

Those who subscribe to the 'conspiracy' theory of government would conclude that this issue is not being dealt with because if there were a national register, it would identify gaps in service which would be expensive to fill. The converse view of the 'cock up' theorists is that the government are not interested anyway, the matter has gone by default or it would not work because of incompetence, and that if anything is to happen, the drive must come from professionals in the field.

There is no doubt in my mind that the greatest shortcoming in the area of promoting the interests of disabled children and their families is the gap between what can be done and what is done. In acute medicine, I think the gap is fairly narrow. In our discipline the standards of care have not on the whole been properly defined, and perhaps we should all try to establish what standards we are capable of achieving. There exist few guidelines for this and I hope that this book will help TDCs to structure their activity, aims and objectives. The goal after this is to do what we say that we do.

REFERENCES

Colver, A.F., Robinson, A. (1989) 'Establishing a register of children with special needs.' *Archives of Disease in Childhood,* **64**, 1200–1203.

Court Report (1976) *Fit for the Future. Report of the Committee on Child Health Services. Vol. 1. Cmnd. 6684.* London: HMSO.

Jolly, H. (1984) 'Have parents the right to see their children's medical reports?' *Archives of Disease in Childhood,* **59**, 601–602.

McConachie, H., Lingam, S., Stiff, B., Holt, K.S. (1988) 'Giving assessment reports to parents.' *Archives of Disease in Childhood,* **63**, 209–210.

Partridge, J.W. (1984) 'Putting it in writing: written assessment reports for parents.' *Archives of Disease in Childhood,* **59**, 678–687.

Weed, L.L. (1968) 'Medical records that guide and teach.' *New England Journal of Medicine,* **278**, 593–600; 652–657.

Woodroffe, C., Abra, A. (1991) 'A special conditions register.' *Archives of Disease in Childhood,* **66**, 927–930.

FURTHER GENERAL BIBLIOGRAPHY

Batshaw, M.L. (1991) *Your Child Has a Disability. A Complete Sourcebook of Daily and Medical Care*. Boston: Little, Brown.

Bleck, E.E. (1987) *Orthopaedic Management in Cerebral Palsy. Clinics in Developmental Medicine No. 99/100*. London: Mac Keith Press.

Darnborough, A., Kinrade, D. (1985) *Directory for Disabled People. A Handbook of Information and Opportunities for Disabled and Handicapped People*. Cambridge: Woodhead-Faulkner in association with RADAR.

Davis, H. (1993) *Counselling Parents of Children with Chronic Illness or Disability*. Leicester: British Psychological Society.

Finnie, N.R. (1974) *Handling the Young Cerebral Palsied Child at Home. 2nd Edn*. London: Heinemann.

Mandelstam, M. (1990) *How to Get Equipment for Disability*. London: Jessica Kingsley.

McCarthy, G.T. (Ed.) *Physical Disability in Childhood. An Interdisciplinary Approach to Management*. Edinburgh: Churchill Livingstone.

Pollack, M. (1993) *Textbook of Developmental Paediatrics*. Edinburgh: Churchill Livingstone.

Polnay, L., Hull, D. (Eds.) (1993) *Community Paediatrics*. Edinburgh: Churchill Livingstone.

Thompson, C.E. (1991) *Raising a Handicapped Child. A Helpful Guide for Parents of the Physically Disabled*. New York: Ballantine.

APPENDIX 1

PLAN OF THE PEMBURY HOSPITAL CHILD DEVELOPMENT CENTRE (CDC)

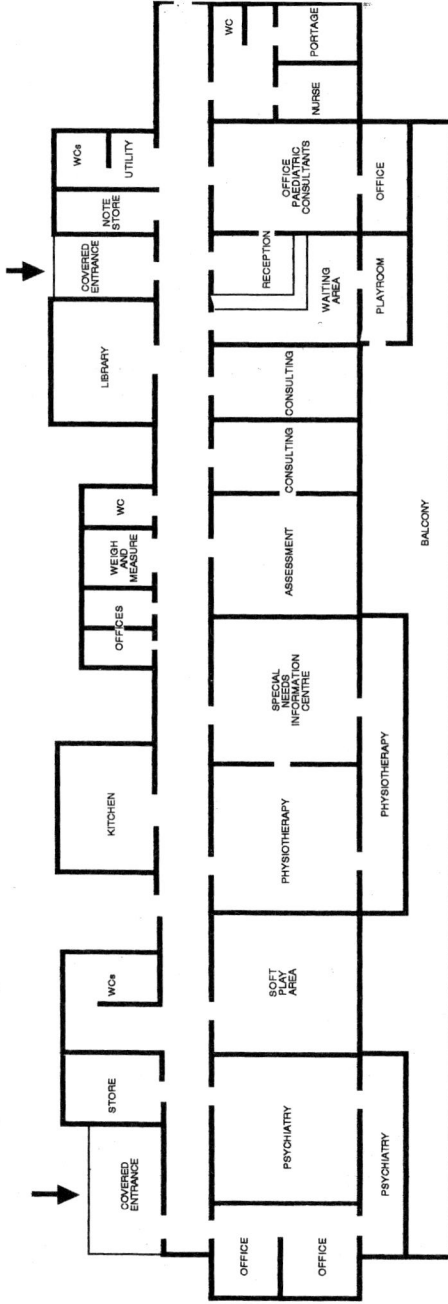

The Pembury Hospital CDC is in a detached building which was modified from an existing paediatric surgical ward. It is all on the ground floor, and only shallow ramps are required for access. When it was modified, some rooms were divided and more indoor space was provided by extending onto the balcony in some places. All the rooms, apart from those on the balcony, are accessible from a common corridor broad enough to allow easy passage for wheelchairs past seats outside consulting rooms. The front of the unit faces south and offers a light aspect. The two covered entrances allow push-chairs etc. to be parked outside if necessary. Fire regulations are fully met. There is generous provision of WCs for both able-bodied and disabled people, children and babies. There is parking space immediately outside, and the unit is well signposted.

APPENDIX 2

A HANDBOOK OF SERVICES FOR CHILDREN WITH SPECIAL NEEDS

A well produced, comprehensive printed guide can be very valuable for the families of children with disabilities. It can also help professionals give quick references on particular issues.

Below are the main topics that need covering. The way they are grouped will vary from place to place, and they are not ranked in any order of importance. They are, however, the issues that most often face professionals dealing with disabled children.

Handbooks of this sort need to be co-ordinated very carefully so that they accurately cover the interests of the various agencies involved. The main focus, however, must always be the reader, and the information given under each of the headings needs to have these factors in mind:

- What entitlements does everyone have?
- What special rights are there for children with disability and their families?
- How can these rights be obtained?
- Where can they be obtained?
- What extra help is available?
- What is special about the local service and how does it differ from others?

Much of the value of the handbook will be in the names and addresses it includes. It is prudent, since these change quite often, to print small quantities and revise frequently. This is more expensive than printing large quantities, but an out-of-date handbook is more nuisance than it is worth. Families with children on the local register of children with disability should be given a copy of each revised issue as it comes out, and the families of all children newly included on the register, whether newcomers from another area or newborn babies, should get a copy automatically.

The main topics are shown below: some of them can be usefully separated for preschool and school-age children.

HEALTH CARE
    Primary Services
        The family doctor
        The district nurse
    Secondary Services (Hospital and Community based)
        In-patient specialist wards in the district
        Out-patient clinics for specific conditions

Team for Disabled Children and their Families (TDC)
Genetic Counselling
Portage Service
Physiotherapy
Hydrotherapy
Dietician
Developmental Assessment
Speech and Language Therapy
Clinical Psychology
Psychiatry
Dental Services
Community Learning Disability Teams (CLDT)

EDUCATION
Preschool Adviser for Children with Special Educational Needs
Hearing Impairment: Services for Children
Visual Impairment: Services for Children
Educational Psychology
Playgroups and Nurseries
    Education Authority Nurseries
    Voluntary Playgroups
Special Schools
Special Units for Children with Specific Disorders
School Health Service

SOCIAL SERVICES - HELP FOR THE FAMILY
Day and Short-Term Care
    Daily child minding
    Holiday playscheme
    Link family scheme
    Short-term residential care
    Emergency care

ADVICE AND SUPPORT
Parent Groups
Support and Information Groups, Local and National
Family Counselling

EQUIPMENT AND AIDS TO LIVING
Feeding, Dressing, Bathing, Bed, Incontinence Aids
Mobility Aids
Adaptations to the Home

ACKNOWLEDGEMENTS

Peter Rosenbaum has not only written a comprehensive and complimentary foreword, but has also provided much appreciated long distance encouragement at each stage of writing. His generous advice and constructive criticism has been a major contribution at a fundamental level.

At Mac Keith Press Martin Bax provided the initial idea and guidance, and I have also quoted freely from his work. Pamela Davies patiently inspired, cajoled and generally motivated the work. Michael Pountney and Pat Chappelle crafted it into a presentable form. Their confidence helped enormously.

Thanks are also due to others whom I have quoted, particularly Lewis Rosenbloom under whose guidance I spent my formative years in child development in Liverpool. Many of his ideas are incorporated, having been assimilated into my practice.

Nearer home I have learnt a great deal from the parents of our patients and hope that this is clear from the text. Special thanks must go to those who allowed me to describe their families and our mutual experiences in detail. I know this was difficult for some and not without pain for them and myself on occasions, and readers will recognise that.

Over the years we have had a very stable team at Pembury, and my thanks go to all those colleagues whom I have worked with and learned from. Their unsung contributions are the essence of the work. We have been well supported regionally by Brian Neville, Richard Robinson and Gillian Baird. My colleague, Wendy Holmes, has been a constant and enthusiastic team member whose role has been central to many of the developments described. Team members, including Nick Anderson, Sue Browne, Liz Critchlow, Liz Elliott, Veronica Fraser, Sheila Minet, Maureen Packwood, Fiona Storrs, Liz Walker and Margaret Williams have all made major contributions.

Finally warm thanks to Elisabeth Jarrett for patience in typing and processing unfamiliar material.

INDEX

Court Report (1976), 2
  child development centre recommendations, 54–55
  on registers, 97
Cystic fibrosis, 34–35

D

Day care nurseries
  Barnado's, 67, 93
  placements, referral, 43
  specialised, 84
Dentato-olivary dysplasia, 11
Developmental delay, 36
Diplegia: hypothetical case, 7–8
Disability
  definition and characteristics, 23
  distinction from handicap, 24
  prevalence, 30
District Handicap Teams (DHTs), 2–3, 55
District Health Authorities, 30
Doman–Delacato therapy, 83
Domiciliary consultation, 65
Donovan, on educational material, 91
Down syndrome, 15–16
  and TDCs, 7
  follow-up, 7
  prevalence, 30
Drooling, Consortium on, 78

E

Early detection of disability, 58–60
Education, 88–93
  assessment venue, 56
  dissatisfaction with, 67
  facilities, 93
  general public, 91
  handbook, 106
  multidisciplinary team, relations with Education Department, 43–44
  notification of special need, statutory, 63
  special needs children, prevalence, 30
Education for All Handicapped Children Act Amendments of 1986 (USA), 80
Empowerment model of consultation, 66–67
Epilepsy, 14–16, 36
Equipment and aids for living, 106
Evered, on liaison psychiatry, 90
Evolution of TDCs, 3–5
Examination, Stone's definition, 28
Expert model of consultation, 63

F

Family
  as consumer of service, 4
  consultation style, 63–67
  factor in early intervention, 79

financial issues, 22, 74, 107
handbook, 90
interaction with team, 9–22
link, 11, 13, 14
multiple-need, 14–19
referral hierarchy, 2
relationship with multidisciplinary team, 41
relationship with professionals, 64–67
  tertiary referral, 70
social network consultation, 65–66
social services, 106
socio-economic factors, 21
stress on, 74
support groups *see* Groups
See also Parents
Ferlie, on 'helping booklet', 90
Financial issues, 22, 74, 107
Fits and hypotonia: hypothetical case, 6
Flesch formula, 61
Follow-up, 68–73
  concomitant appointments, 68
  location, 68
Forming, of multidisciplinary team, 49
Foundation for Conductive Education, Birmingham, 83
Function limitation, prevalence, 30
Fund-raising, 92
Future prospects: consultation with parent, 62

G

Gait analysis, 8
Gale and Grant, on medical change, 51, 52
General practitioners, role in education, 89
Genetic counselling
  cerebral palsy, 16
  diplegia, 8
  following early diagnosis, 60
Genetic factors, 63
Graduation to adult services, 45, 72–73
Grieving process, 9, 71
Groups, 85
  self-help, 45, 46, 91, 106
Growth/intellectual development, 25
'Gunning fog' test of readability, 91

H

Hall, on screening and surveillance, 26, 60
Handbook for families, 90
Handbook of Early Childhood Intervention (Meisels and Shonkoff), 80
Handbook for services for children with special needs: guidelines, 105–107
Handicap
  definition and characteristics, 23–24
  distinction from disability, 24
  socio-educational aspect, 25

110

O

Occupational therapy, 76, 79
Office of Population Censuses and Surveys, report on disability, 30
Ontario, prevalence of disability, 30
Osteogenesis imperfecta, 18–19
O'Sullivan, on parent satisfaction, 76
Otosclerosis, 19
'Over-structuring', dangers of, 4

P

Paediatrician as primary health carer, 58
Parents
  as therapists, 76, 77
    See also Portage
  consultation styles, 63–67
  expectations, 62
  note-holding, 72, 95
  relationship with professionals, 2
  relationship with team, 41
  role in education, 90–91
  satisfaction, 76
  self-help, *see* Groups
  therapeutic needs, 74–76
  See also Family
Partridge, on children's notes, 96
Patients' Charter, The, 64
Payment for services, 65
Pearson, on the multidisciplinary team, 46–47
Pembury Hospital Child Development Centre, 104
Performing, of the multidisciplinary team, 49
Peto Institute, Budapest, 83
Physiotherapy, 77
Portage, 10, 14 *et seq.*, 63, 77, 81–83
  groups, 85
  parent representation, 66
  speech and language disorder, 78
  toy libraries, 84
Postviral fatigue syndrome (myalgic encephalo-myelitis), 25
Poverty, and chronic health problems, *see* Socio-economic aspects
Primary care team, 58
  education, 89
Professional hierarchies, 46
Progressive neurological disease, 10
Psychiatrist, child, in the multidisciplinary team, 41
Psychiatry, liaison, 44, 90
Psychologist, in the multidisciplinary team, 41
Psychomotor problems, registration, 36
Public awareness, 91–93
Pulmonary hypertension, 15

R

Rare disabilities, referral, 70
Records, *see* Notes

Reed, pre-consultation recommendations, 61
Referral, 58–61
  by colleagues, awareness of, 36
  further, 69
  hierarchy, 1
  in the multidisciplinary team, 41
  monitoring, 60
  outside the district, 69–70
  rare disabilities, 70
  responsibility within the team, 4
  sources, 58
  tertiary education activities, 89
Reforming, of the multidisciplinary team, 49
Registers, 97–102
  need for national system, 101
  uses, 101
Registration
  and monitoring, 39
  of special needs, 36
Rehabilitation schools, 72
Research Trust for Metabolic Disease in Children, 45, 91
Responsibility for patient, 3
Richmond, on early intervention, 79
Role of TDC, 5
Role release, 48
Rosenbaum, on home assessment, 55
Rosenbloom and Marlow, on training (medical students and junior staff), 89

S

Scandinavia, prevalence of health problems in, 30–32
Scope of work of TDCs, 6–9
Screening, 26–29, 60
  Stone's definition, 27–28
Scrutton, on aim orientated management, 78
Second (and third) opinion, 70–72
Self-help groups *see* Groups
Sensory neural hearing loss, early detection, 60
Sex differences, in prevalence of disability, 32
Social services
  and the multidisciplinary team, 45
  consultation model, 65–66
  handbook, 106
Social worker, and the multidisciplinary team, 41
Socioeconomic aspects of family coping, 21
Soft play areas, 85
Sotos syndrome, 25
Spastic diplegia, 17–19
Special investigations: consultation with parent, 62
Specialised clinics, TDC, 69
Specialist visitors, training, 70
Speech and language therapy, 77, 78
Staff development approach, 48
'Statementing', 44, 63, 85

NOTES

NOTES

NOTES

Department of Child Health
The Queen's University of Belfast